W9-DIJ-022

The Ultimate Detox
Dr Cabot, Sandra & Margaret Jasinska ND

First published 2005 by WHAS
P. O. Box 689 Camden NSW 2570 Australia
02 4655 8855
www.whas.com.au

First Edition printed January 2005

Categories
1.Detox. 2. Cleansing 3. Diet. 4. Toxins 5. Nutrition. 6. Women's Health Advisory Service

Disclaimer
The suggestions, ideas and treatments described in this book must not replace the care and direct supervision of a trained health care professional. All problems and concerns regarding your health require medical supervision. If you have any pre-existing medical disorders, you must consult your own doctor before following the suggestions in this book. If you are taking any prescribed medications you should check with your own doctor before using the recommendations in this book.

Printed by Griffin Press
Typeset by Christopher Martin
Illustrations by Christopher Martin

ISBN: 0-958-61373-7

www.whas.com.au
www.weightcontroldoctor.com
www.liverdoctor.com

CONTENTS

Contents

CONTENTS

Subject	Page

About the Authors

Dr Sandra Cabot MBBS, DRCOG,

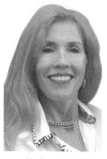

Dr Sandra Cabot is a medical doctor who has extensive clinical experience; she treats patients with hormonal imbalances, chronic diseases and weight problems.

Dr Cabot works with other medical doctors and her team of naturopaths; her practices are situated in Camden and Broadway, Sydney, NSW.

Dr Sandra Cabot began studying nutritional medicine while she was a medical student and has been a pioneer in the area of holistic healing. She graduated in medicine with honours from the University of Adelaide, South Australia in 1975. During the1980s Dr Cabot worked as a volunteer in the largest missionary Christian hospital in India, tending to the poor indigenous women.

Dr Cabot pilots herself to many cities and country towns in Australia where she is invited to speak at seminars and exhibitions. Feel free to direct any questions to our online help at www.whas.com.au

Margaret Jasinska ND, DBM

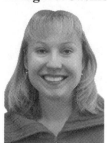

Margaret Jasinska is a naturopath who has been in clinical practice for seven years and now works very closely on a day to day basis with Dr Sandra Cabot. Margaret has a particular interest in disorders of the digestive and immune systems. She has researched environmental medicine encompassing the effects of environmental chemicals on health and disease.

Margaret is a keen researcher and writer, and enjoys keeping abreast of new developments in the health industry. She is currently working with Dr Cabot on a book about cholesterol.

Margaret enjoys helping individuals improve their health through dietary modification and nutritional medicine.

Margaret is available for consultations at the Dr Sandra Cabot Holistic Health Clinic in Camden ph (02) 4655 4666.

I am a firm believer in the value of supporting the detoxification systems in the body especially in this day and age, where mankind has disturbed the natural environment and the food chain. The fact that we are exposed to more toxic chemicals and rapidly spread infections than ever before, is unquestionable.

I see many patients with disorders of their immune system and liver who have been unable to get an accurate diagnosis or effective treatment from drug therapy. These patients find that a so called "healthy conventional diet" does not improve their health. So what are these patients to do? Surely they do not want to give up in their search for a solution and accept a life of poor health!

If you are in this situation, I would encourage you to try a safe and effective detoxification program, such as you will find in this book. I think it is a great idea to use regular detox strategies everyday, even if you are in relatively good health, as a preventative measure to keep your immune system strong. This includes juicing of raw vegetables, as this provides a high concentration of antioxidants to support the liver detoxification pathways. You can also include the specific foods and supplements mentioned in the body of this book on a regular basis in your daily life to keep your immune system strong. There is a huge body of evidence available to show that those who consume a diet high in fresh fruits and vegetables and take antioxidants such as selenium, zinc, vitamin C and vitamin E have a stronger immune system.

Still there are detractors out there who heap scorn on the virtues of detoxification diets and cleansing diets, saying that they are useless or even dangerous. So let us examine their arguments against the value of detoxification diets.

1 Many of these diets prescribe a huge intake of water of up to 4 to 5 litres daily. If they do, they are too fanatical, as excess water intake, especially if combined with fasting, can cause an imbalance in the concentration of sodium in the body, which is called hyponatraemia. It is true that sodium deficiency can lead to swelling of the brain and coma and convulsions. So be wary of fanatical detoxification diets that tell you to drink more than 3 litres of water daily with ONLY raw fruits and vegetables. I am not advocating that.

2 Some of these detoxification programs excessively restrict the intake of protein and carbohydrates, which may disrupt metabolism resulting in low levels of albumin in the blood stream and unstable blood sugar levels. Our 2-week detoxification diet is nutritionally balanced and provides you with adequate protein and carbohydrate.

3 Detox diets are always dangerous. This is not true, as they should be temporary and they are far safer than a diet high in sugar, fried take away foods, refined processed foods and alcohol. However if you are pregnant, breastfeeding, very underweight, diabetic or suffer with any chronic medical illness you should NOT follow ANY detoxification diet. You should always consult your own doctor in such cases.

4 Some detractors say that your liver and kidneys are able to detoxify your body without any help from you, which assumes that they are always working at 100% efficiency. This is not always true. For example if you have a fatty liver where the liver's filter is overloaded with fat, bacteria and toxins, it will not cleanse the blood stream efficiently. Like any filter in any engine, the liver filter needs cleansing, and unfortunately you cannot unzip your abdomen and take out your liver and wash it with running water and a degreasing agent! Nearly 20% of the population has a fatty liver because of years of incorrect diet and damage from drugs and environmental toxins. Many drugs and environmental toxins over work the natural detoxification pathways and filtering mechanisms in the liver and kidneys. This is one of the reasons that unexplained liver and kidney disease is so common.

Infections in the body (either hidden or apparent infections) can cause diseases of the kidneys and heart, so obviously in such cases, the natural detox and defense systems in the body were not functioning at 100% of their capacity. If the infection is resistant to antibiotics or anti-viral drugs, your only hope lies in bolstering your natural immune defenses and detoxification pathways. Infections release toxins that your body needs help to deal with; if not these infections would never cause diseases.

5 ALL detoxification diets are fanatical and based on extreme ideas of restriction. An example of such extremes would be prolonged fasting on raw juices only, or a water only diet, or eating only one type of food (such as offal or grapes or grapefruits), or the infamous "Breatharian Diet," which advocated nothing but fresh air! Well I am not advocating these extreme approaches and indeed I think fasting is potentially dangerous, especially in those who have medical problems or those who have had a very toxic lifestyle with excess intake of alcohol, cigarettes and junk food. The resultant rapid release of toxins induced by a strict juicing fast would result in unpleasant and potentially dangerous symptoms. However if you look at most of the detox diets advocated by naturopaths and nutritionists you would find that they are not extreme and indeed are well balanced. I think if the protagonist or author of the detox diet is well qualified in the science of nutrition and medicine that their ideas would be well balanced.

6 Your metabolism will slow down on a detox diet because it is deficient in nutrients and calories, and thus when you come off it, and start to eat normally, you will put on weight more rapidly than ever before. In other words these detractors say that detox diets are fattening! Well my experiences are to the contrary and many of my overweight patients have found that they lose weight for the first time in years, just because they have introduced greater amounts of cleansing and raw foods into their diet. They did not reduce their intake of calories. Indeed I had one patient who lost over 10 kilograms just by starting to do raw juicing and eating one salad a day. This was because the raw foods improved the ability of her liver to burn fat.

7 Detox diets play on the vulnerability of those with eating disorders such as anorexia and bulimia. I disagree with this, as these patients often follow extreme diets where they eat massive amounts of any types of foods and then purge themselves with laxatives, emetics and diuretics. We are not advocating that patients take these types of drugs. These patients are vulnerable to nutritional deficiencies because they either avoid all types of food or try to expel the food from their bodies after ingesting it. These patients need counseling and sometimes medication and are generally looking to lose enormous amounts of weight rather than to detox themselves.

8 Detox diets are very narrowly focused and ignore exercise and stress management. Well remember a safe detox diet is only temporary, and if you feel tired, it's not good to force yourself to sweat it out in the gym. If you feel well while detoxing, I encourage you to do some gentle exercising such as walking, swimming and yoga. Exercise can help the detox process because it promotes the flow of lymphatic fluid, which carries the peripheral toxins away from the tissues. Exercise also helps you to sweat more, which helps the elimination of toxins through the skin. For the same reasons saunas and body brushing can help, but remember you do not have to put your body under extreme measures of any of these modalities to achieve a detoxing benefit. Stress management can help in the detoxification process because excess stress causes the release of too much adrenalin and cortisol from the adrenal glands and this can have toxic effects. Good techniques of stress management are positive affirmations, mediation, prayer, massage and talking to close friends who believe in you. They can help you to stick to your path and believe in your own abilities.

9 To those who disparage all forms of detoxing and cleansing, I would ask what is their clinical experience in helping patients who have tried every conventional treatment going, including the so called "healthy diet"? Believe me, the term "healthy diet" means one hundred different things to a hundred different professionals. They all have their own fixed ideas and today there is so much disagreement between "dietary experts". There are still those who believe in low fat, which goes against the theory of the low-carb protagonists, whilst others still say to their patients that their diet is not of great importance and that medication is the controlling factor in success.

Let me share a case history with you, which demonstrates the therapeutic value of detoxing. One of my patients presented to me for the first time in a terrible state. She had a bright purple psychedelic rash all over her face. This rash had been caused by the antibiotic drugs she had been prescribed to treat her mature onset acne. This type of acne is known as acne rosacea. The antibiotic had not only caused this rash, it had also caused acute liver inflammation. The well meaning dermatologist had then prescribed this woman cortisone to suppress the side effects of the antibiotic. Unfortunately the cortisone damaged her heart resulting in an irregular heart beat. When I saw the patient I diagnosed a fatty liver, which was seen on her ultrasound scan, and also explained why she was overweight and had developed the inflammatory acne in the first place. I placed her on the Liver Cleansing Diet and gave her a cleansing liver tonic and a program of raw vegetable juicing. Within 3 months she had lost 12 kilograms, her face was now completely free of acne and the purple rash had gone and her liver function was normal. I have many case histories like this, and thus I am talking with the conviction of clinical experience in helping patients who are often looking for a last resort.

Effective detoxing is not only for the rich and self-pampered and you don't need to spend thousands of dollars at expensive health retreats and spas if you cannot afford it. You will find that our 2-week detox-plan is easy and inexpensive to follow. Furthermore if you have questions or problems while following this 2-week detox plan, you can get free help. To get more help you may call the Health Advisory Service on 02 4655 8855 or email help@whas.com.au

Living in today's world, detoxification has never been so relevant. Whether we like it or not, we are continually exposed to an array of ever increasing chemicals. Therefore, now more than ever we must ensure we are as healthy as possible, in order to cope in this toxic world.

It has been estimated there are approximately 100 000 toxic waste dumps in Australia. Most of these were filled with a soup of discarded chemicals many years ago. A lot of these chemicals would have leached into groundwater. The problem is that as the urban sprawl continues to spread, new housing developments are built on former landfills, bunkers and industrial sites of the past. Ref. 1.

As the environment becomes more and more polluted, so do our bodies.

The major detoxification systems of the body comprise the liver, kidneys, bowels, lymphatic system, spleen, lungs and skin. In an ideal world, these systems work together to rid our bodies of the toxins produced within, as a by-product of metabolism, and the toxins that have entered our body from the outside world.

However, pollution, toxins, stress and a less than perfect diet, leading to nutritional deficiencies, place a greater load on our body's detoxification abilities. Over time, our body's ability to rid itself of toxins becomes poorer, and the toxins start to accumulate in our tissues. This places an enormous stress on our immune system. Immune disorders are one of the fastest growing group of diseases. Allergies, food intolerances, autoimmune diseases and chronic infections are on a steep climb.

To assist your body in being a better detoxifier, your day to day diet and lifestyle are the most important factors. There is little benefit to eating like a Buddhist monk for two weeks out of the year, and like a child at an amusement park the rest of the time, thinking that you'll undo the damage. Prevention is better than cure, and it is best to minimise your exposure to toxins and chemicals as much as you can. Many of the chemicals we are exposed to these days, whether they are in food or the environment are newly created molecules that take very many years to break down. This means our body really hasn't developed a strategy to deal with these chemicals. Preventing exposure to them is really your best option, because once they have entered your body it may be too late.

What we aim to do with this two week detoxification diet is to give you a kick start to improving your health, and to make you take a long hard look at the kinds of foods you regularly eat. Are they helping or harming you? We want you to start feeling better, be more energetic, lose some weight, have clearer skin and prevent degenerative diseases. Once you are feeling better about your health, and yourself, this may inspire you to continue paying more attention to your diet. We also want to make you aware of the many choices you have in your life; we are not advocating you pack up your belongings, move out of the city and set up camp in a pristine forest. That would drastically reduce your toxic exposure, no doubt. However, just by being more aware of the kinds of chemicals you use in your home, and the kind of pots and pans you cook your food in, you can already make huge improvements.

The Ultimate Detox

Chapter One

WHY DETOX?

What Are The Benefits Of Detoxification?

By following our two week eating plan, and continuing with the healthy eating principles, you can experience a number of health benefits, such as:

*   Achieving a healthy weight
*   Increased energy
*   Reduced cravings

- Clearer skin
- Less frequent and severe headaches
- Less indigestion
- Improved bowel habits – less constipation or irritable bowel syndrome
- Have a sharper mind and better memory
- Improved liver function
- Improved immune system
- Better moods – less anxiety and depression
- Better sleep
- Reduce the effects of ageing
- Balanced hormones – less PMS, menstrual cramps and an easier menopause
- Less fluid retention and bloating
- A healthy libido
- A healthier pregnancy and baby

Chapter Two

THE BODY'S DETOXIFICATION SYSTEMS AND HOW THEY WORK

What Are The Detoxification Systems Of The Body and How Do They Work?

Because our body is continually exposed to toxins, in one form or another, our body is constantly trying to remove toxins. The liver is the chief detoxification organ in your body. Every toxin you are exposed to, whether it is something you ate, inhaled, or rubbed onto your skin; all these chemicals will arrive at your liver.

However, the liver has a lot of help from other organs and body systems, and the liver only really converts the toxins into a form that is more easily excreted by other organs .

None of the detoxification systems below work in isolation; they are all intimately linked and depend on each other. So you can't just do a liver detox for instance, and not affect other parts of your body.

If one detox system is overworked or overburdened, this will place additional stress on another system. Let's now look at them one by one.

The Liver
Structure of the Liver

The liver is the largest internal organ in our body, and weighs approximately 1.36kg (3 pounds). It is located in the upper right quadrant of the abdomen. It is divided into two major lobes; right and left, and two minor lobes; caudate and quadrate. The right and left lobes are separated by fibrous tissue called the falciform ligament.

The inferior surface or underside of the liver contains a kind of gate called a porta. This is where veins, arteries, nerves and lymphatic vessels enter and leave the liver. The hepatic ducts are what transport bile out of the liver; the right and left hepatic ducts join to form a common hepatic duct. This unites with the cystic duct from the gallbladder to form the common bile duct. It is through this duct that bile enters the small intestine.
Walls of connective tissue divide the liver into hexagon-shaped lobules with a portal triad at each corner. They are called triads because three vessels are located in them. Hepatic cords radiate out from the central vein of each lobule like spokes of a wheel. Hepatic cords are made of hepatocytes (liver cells). Between these

rows of liver cells there are spaces called sinusoids. The sinusoids are lined with special cells such as fat storing cells, endothelial cells, pit cells, and Kupffer cells.

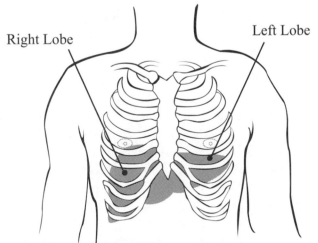

Right Lobe

Left Lobe

Location of the Liver in the body

Kupffer cells are an interesting kind of immune cell. They behave like Pac Man and have the ability to engulf, devour and destroy toxins. Kupffer cells are mobile; they travel around the sinusoids and ingest dead cells, cancer cells, bacteria, parasites, yeasts, viruses, artificial chemicals and other foreign particles. So obviously, the better your Kupffer cells are working, the fewer toxins will escape into your bloodstream and enter other tissues.

The liver is a very important organ in our body. It performs at least 500 known functions, and generates a large amount of heat in the body. That is why people with an overworked liver may feel excessively hot or perspire profusely. The liver is the only organ in the body that receives a double blood supply. It receives oxygen-rich blood from the heart and lungs via the hepatic artery, and oxygen-depleted, but nutrient rich blood from the intestines via the portal vein. Therefore, the first stop of blood from the digestive tract is the liver. The greater the amount of toxins in the digestive tract, the more toxins will enter the liver. If the liver becomes overwhelmed with toxins, they can then enter the bloodstream, and organs.

What Are The Major Functions Of The Liver?

• **Carbohydrate, protein and fat metabolism:** The liver converts glucose into glycogen for storage. When blood sugar levels fall, (between meals), the glycogen can be re-converted into glucose again to raise blood sugar levels. The liver also produces glucose tolerance factor from chromium and other nutrients. This works with insulin to regulate blood sugar levels. Therefore, diabetics wishing to have better control of their blood sugar must ensure they have a healthy liver.

The liver is also where the majority of triglycerides and cholesterol are manufactured; hence your blood levels of these fats are largely dependant on your liver function.

• **Hormone metabolism:** The liver is the major site of hormone breakdown. Hormones, such as oestrogen are secreted into the bile and enter the small intestine for excretion. If the liver is overworked, symptoms of oestrogen dominance such as PMS, menstrual cramps and swollen, lumpy breasts may result. Inefficient breakdown of androgens (male hormones) may produce symptoms such as acne, scalp hair loss and excessive facial hair in women. If your bowel is sluggish you will not excrete these hormones properly; they will be reabsorbed in your intestines, recirculate and lead to higher blood levels.

The thyroid hormone T4 (thyroxine) is converted into its active form T3 (tri-iodothyronine) in the liver. Sex Hormone Binding Globulin (SHBG) is manufactured in the liver; this carries hormones such as oestrogen and testosterone around our bloodstream.

• **Digestive functions:** The liver manufactures approximately 600 to 1000mL of bile each day. Bile is necessary for fat digestion, as it emulsifies fat; that is, it breaks down fat globules into smaller bits so that it may be absorbed. Bile is the major route for the excretion of a number of substances including:

> *cholesterol and other fats
> *bilirubin (resulting from the breakdown of haemoglobin)
> *fat soluble hormones
> *toxins broken down by the liver

Once secreted into the intestines, these substances can be absorbed by fibre from our diet and excreted out in bowel motions. If we do not consume enough fibre, toxins and cholesterol can be reabsorbed back into our bloodstream.

• **Storage of vitamins and minerals:** Vitamins A, D, B12, K and E are stored in the liver, along with copper and iron. Enough of these can be stored to last several months. The liver also converts vitamin D into its active form, needed for calcium metabolism.

• **Detoxification:** The liver is able to detoxify many toxic substances that enter our body; it alters their structure, making them less toxic, or more easily excreted. Inside the hepatocytes, enzyme systems are capable of breaking down, or metabolising drugs, chemicals, hormones, pesticides and other toxins. The majority of chemicals entering our body are fat soluble, or lipophilic (fat loving). This means that they may be stored in fatty tissues such as the brain, cell membranes and our body fat stores. It is the liver's job to convert these toxins into water soluble chemicals, so that they may be excreted in watery fluids such as urine, bile and sweat.

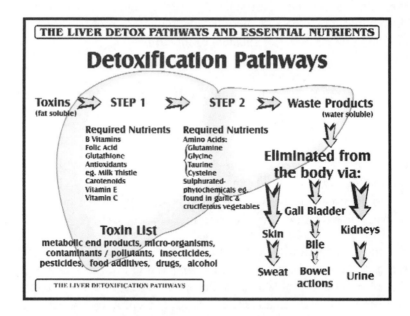

Phase One Detoxification

Phase one is carried out mainly by a group of enzymes called **cytochrome P 450s**. The function of these enzymes is **biotransformation**; this means the metabolic conversion of xenobiotics (foreign chemicals), hormones and fatty acids into a more active form. This is achieved through a number of chemical reactions including oxidation, reduction, hydrolysis, dehalogenation and hydration.

These enzymes are greatly affected by dietary, environmental and lifestyle factors. Hence, there is great variation among people in their ability to biotransform toxins.

These processes tend to generate a lot of free radicals, which have the potential to damage our liver cells. This is because the end products of phase one detoxification (called reactive intermediates), are usually more harmful and destructive than the original molecule. Reactive intermediates can wreck a lot of havoc in our bodies; they act as free radicals and may cause direct damage to cells and DNA, and irritate the immune system.

This means that we must have plenty of antioxidants available to our liver cells, to mop up these free radicals. It is important for the phase two detoxification pathway to work well, so that these chemicals do not hang around in our liver cells for long.

Phase Two Detoxification

This phase involves conjugation reactions, whereby another substance is added to a toxin, to make it less harmful. The various conjugation reactions include the following:
*   Glutathione conjugation
*   Sulphation
*   Methylation
*   Acetylation
*   Glycination
*   Amino acid conjugation

This process makes the toxin more water soluble, so that it is easier to excrete. For efficient phase two detoxification, ample amounts of sulphur bearing amino acids such as cysteine and taurine are required. Glycine, glutamine, choline and inositol are also needed in adequate quantities. The phase two enzyme systems utilise large amounts of glutathione. This is the most powerful antioxidant and liver protector in our body.

Ideally phase one and two reactions should occur in a rapidly co-ordinated action.
If we are exposed to a large amount of toxins, and/or we are deficient in the co-factors needed for detoxification to occur; a build-up of toxins will result. This means a large amount of toxins will spill into the bloodstream. Over time it can lead to hyper-

stimulation and exhaustion of the immune system. This may result in a tendency to develop allergies, autoimmune conditions or repeated infections.

Functional Liver Detoxification Tests

A liver function test is a standard blood test which may be ordered by a GP to measure the blood levels of various liver enzymes, bilirubin and blood proteins. Unfortunately this test is not very sensitive, and can only detect whether there is actual liver disease present. You may have a normal liver function test result, yet still have significant liver dysfunction.

There are more specific tests that can be used to assess the liver's detoxification abilities; these tests are referred to as a Comprehensive Detoxification Profile test, or a Functional Liver Detoxification Profile. These tests involve challenging the liver with safe oral doses of caffeine, paracetamol and aspirin. Samples of urine and saliva are collected at specifically timed intervals; these are sent to a laboratory which measures the levels of the breakdown products of these drugs.

These tests determine the ability of the liver to detoxify and eliminate drugs and chemicals. They specifically assess both phase one and phase two detoxification pathways by the liver. These tests can be ordered by your doctor, naturopath or nutritionist and you can conduct them in your own home. Results are sent to a laboratory for assessment.

Benefits of These Tests

Our bodies are continually exposed to environmental chemicals and toxins produced in our own body. These tests reflect the degree we are exposed to toxins, and our body's ability to deal with them.

If phase one and phase two detoxification are out of balance, free radicals build up and can create damage to tissues. Most commonly phase one is adequate or overactive, and phase two is sluggish. These tests can let you find out if this is happening in your body.

Deficiencies of various vitamins, minerals or amino acids can slow down specific steps in phase one or two detoxification. These tests enable you to find out exactly which nutrients are lacking in your diet, and how this is affecting your liver's ability to detoxify. The two main laboratories offering these functional liver tests are:

• Analytical Reference Laboratories Pty Ltd
www.arlaus.com.au
Phone (03) 9529 2922

• Great Smokies Diagnostic Laboratory
www.gsdl.com
Phone (828)253-0621 This lab is in the USA

The Intestines

Nutritional medicine places a great emphasis on the digestive tract. This is understandable because it is where we obtain the goodness from the food we eat; and where we excrete toxins which would be harmful to our bodies if left to remain. The health of our liver, lymphatic system and immune system are greatly affected by the state of our intestines.

How Our Digestive System Works

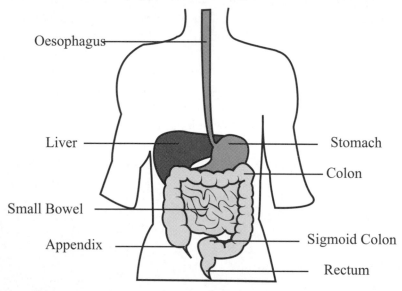

Digestion begins in the mouth, where food is chewed, mixed with saliva and swallowed. So bolting your food down in a hurry isn't a good start to healthy digestion. We produce approximately 1 to 1.5 litres of saliva daily. The saliva contains some enzymes that begin carbohydrate digestion, lysozymes (substances with an antibacterial action), and IgA; also antibacterial.

The stomach acts mainly to churn and store food. Its surface is covered by a thick, protective layer of mucus; helping to protect it from damage caused by hydrochloric acid and enzymes. Parietal cells of the stomach produce intrinsic factor; this binds with vitamin B12 and enhances its absorption in the small intestine. The hydrochloric acid produced by the stomach lowers the pH to between 1 and 3. This low pH helps to kill off a lot of bacteria that we inevitably ingest on our food and fingers. It also activates the protein digesting enzymes in our stomach. It is mainly protein that gets digested in our stomach, and food usually stays in there for between three and four hours. Contractions of the stomach produce hunger pangs, and occur as a result of an empty stomach or a fall in blood sugar levels. Therefore, keeping your blood sugar level stable is a good way to avoid excessive hunger.

The small intestine is where digestion is completed, and most absorption occurs here. There are three segments that make up the small intestine: the duodenum, jejunum and ileum. Bile from the gallbladder and digestive juices from the pancreas enter the duodenum through an opening called Vater's ampulla. A ring of muscle called the sphincter of Oddi controls the opening and closing of the ampulla. The intestinal lining also produces digestive enzymes. This is important to remember because if it is inflamed or ulcerated, these enzymes cannot be produced, so food will not be digested properly.

In order to maximise absorption in the small intestine, its lining contains a number of folds called **villi**. These look a lot like a shag-pile carpet. Each villus contains blood capillaries, and a lymph capillary called a lacteal. Digested fats are absorbed into the lacteals, and transported in the lymph, whereas all other absorbed substances enter the blood capillaries and are taken to the liver. A system of blood vessels called the hepatic portal system transports blood from the intestine to the liver. Therefore the first stop of all blood from your intestines is the liver. So you can see that a toxic bowel will quickly lead to a toxic liver. The reabsorption of bile salts, fat and toxins from the bowel wall to the liver is called the entero-hepatic circulation.

The large intestine consists of the colon and rectum. The colon begins with the caecum; a pouch from where the appendix attaches. The colon then has an ascending, transverse and descending portion. From there it becomes the sigmoid colon, which joins the rectum. It takes food 18 to 24 hours to pass along the entire length of the colon. The main functions of the large intestines are:
 --the formation and excretion of faeces
 -- the absorption of water and minerals,
 --beneficial bacteria in the colon manufacture vitamins B1, B2, B12 and vitamin K. They also help to prevent the overgrowth of

harmful bacteria.

Cells of the colon secrete mucus which lubricates and protects the walls. Inflammation or irritation of the intestinal wall causes the release of large amounts of mucus, as well as water and electrolytes. In this case mucus can be seen in the stools, and there may be diarrhoea.

On the other hand, if faeces remain in the colon for longer than desirable, causing constipation, large amounts of toxins will be reabsorbed back into the bloodstream. This is called auto-intoxication, or self poisoning.

The Urinary System

The urinary system consists of two bean-shaped kidneys, which are roughly the size of clenched fists; two ureters, which transport urine to the bladder, and a urethra, which takes urine out of the body.

The kidneys receive toxins that have been broken down and made water soluble by the liver; such as the end products of medications, organic chemicals, yeast, and hormones. The breakdown products of protein digestion; urea and ammonia are also excreted by the kidneys.

Our kidneys sit on either side of the spine, at the mid-lower back. The right kidney sits slightly lower than the left kidney, because of the presence of the liver above it. Approximately 1176mL of blood passes through our kidneys each minute, and a healthy person produces between one and two litres of urine each day.

The functional unit of the kidneys is called the nephron. There are around 1, 300, 000 nephrons in each kidney. Blood is filtered through a knot of capillaries into the cup-shaped Bowman's capsule. From here, water and many other substances pass into the renal tubule. Most substances are reabsorbed back into the blood;

the remaining fluid becomes urine and drains into the ureters and enters the bladder. Urine gets its yellow colour from compounds in bile from the liver.

The kidneys maintain a constant balance of water and minerals in the blood. We also lose water through the breath, intestinal tract and skin. It is our kidney's job to make sure our fluid and electrolyte levels remain consistent each day. If you don't consume much fluid during the day, you will produce little urine, which is concentrated and darkly coloured. In hot climates or intense physical exertion your urine output will also be less, as you lose more water through your skin in perspiration.

Having clear or faintly yellow urine is better than a strong yellow, concentrated urine because it reduces your chances of developing kidney stones. The more concentrated the urine, the greater the chance that minerals in the urine will form stones. If you do not produce much urine, toxins will have to leave your body through other avenues, such as the bowels, skin and perspiration. Taking B vitamins can colour your urine bright yellow due to riboflavin (vitamin B2).

The Lymphatic System

The lymphatic system consists of the following: lymph, lymphocytes, lymph vessels, lymph nodes, tonsils, the thymus gland, Peyer's patches of the intestines, and the spleen. Fluids move out of our blood capillaries, into tissue spaces, and then enter lymph capillaries. The fluid that enters these capillaries is called lymph. Lympha means water, and this describes the clear, colourless appearance of the fluid. We actually have approximately three times the amount of lymph fluid in our bodies as we do blood.
Lymph capillaries join to form larger lymph vessels. Blood is pumped around our body by the heart's contractions, but that is

not the case with lymph. Most of the time lymphatic fluid flows against gravity. Three factors help to keep it moving:

--contractions of surrounding skeletal muscles during exercise or daily activities. This can increase
  lymph flow by as much as 10 to 15 times.

--contractions of smooth muscle in the lymph vessel walls.

--movements of the chest during breathing.

So just by increasing your activity level and breathing deeply, you will be cleansing your lymphatic system.

There are many lymph nodes located along the lymph vessels. They function as collection sites, and lymph must pass through them before it enters the blood. Eventually lymph vessels join to form either the right or left subclavian vein. Vessels from the right arm, right side of the head and neck enter the right lymphatic duct. Lymph vessels from the rest of the body enter the thoracic duct. From here lymph enters the general circulation.

The lymphatic system performs three main functions:

--It maintains fluid balance in the body. Substances in blood such as nutrients, gases, some protein and ions leave blood capillaries and become part of the lymph. Also substances inside cells such as waste products, hormones and enzymes enter lymphatic fluid.

--It absorbs fats from the digestive tract through vessels called lacteals. These are found in the lining of the small intestine. Due to its fat content, lymph here has a milky appearance.

--It acts like a garbage collection service. It filters the bloodstream of toxins and wastes. Lymph nodes contain large amounts of white blood cells that engulf bacteria. If we have an infection, the nodes closest to the site enlarge because many white blood cells multiply inside them. This enlargement of the lymph nodes can make them sore and tender.

Let's take a closer look at some of the organs of the lymphatic system:

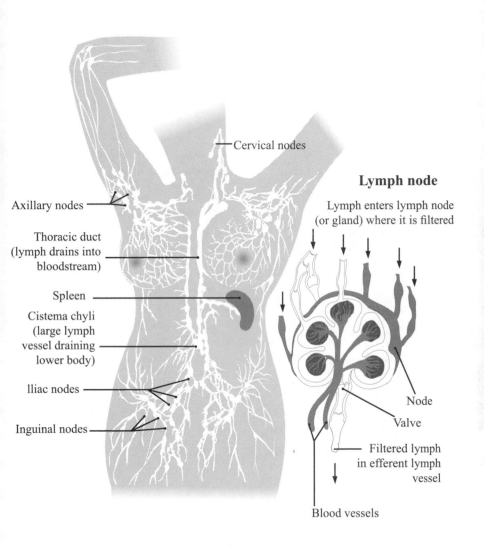

Cervical nodes

Lymph node

Lymph enters lymph node
(or gland) where it is filtered

Axillary nodes

Thoracic duct
(lymph drains into
bloodstream)

Spleen

Cistema chyli
(large lymph
vessel draining
lower body)

lliac nodes

Inguinal nodes

Node

Valve

Filtered lymph
in efferent lymph
vessel

Blood vessels

Components of the Lymphatic System

GALT

GALT stands for Gut Associated Lymphoid Tissue. As the name implies, it is found in the intestines and comprises of lymphocytes, macrophages, Peyer's patches and lymph nodes. GALT is considered the largest collection of immune cells in the body. 70 percent of all antibody producing cells in the body are located in the GALT. Ref. 2.

You probably didn't know that the most important part of your immune system is in your gut!

The GALT works hard to prevent unwanted micro organisms such as bacteria, viruses, fungi, yeast and parasites from entering our body.

The Spleen

The spleen is located high up on the left side of the abdomen, and is around the size of a clenched fist. It has two main functions:

--It filters blood through channels called sinuses. Red blood cells squeeze through these channels, and older, worn out cells are destroyed there.

--It assists the immune system by producing large amounts of white blood cells called lymphocytes which help to fight infections.

The spleen is protected by the ribs, but it is a soft organ, so is easily ruptured through injuries such as occurring from car accidents or contact sports. Sometimes the spleen will need to be removed (splenectomy). In this case the liver and other lymphatic tissues compensate for its functions.

The Lungs

The lungs lie on either side of the heart, in the chest cavity. Each lung is roughly the shape of a pyramid, with the bases sitting on top of the diaphragm. Gas exchange is the main function of our lungs; inhaled oxygen is supplied to the blood, and carbon dioxide is exhaled. The lungs are divided into lobes; there are usually three

in the right lung, and two in the left lung.
To reach the lungs, air enters the trachea, which then divides into two main bronchi. The bronchi divide repeatedly into smaller and smaller tubes called bronchioles. These in turn subdivide into tiny clusters of air sacs called alveoli. These alveoli have a very rich blood supply, so any chemical you inhale can reach your bloodstream via your lungs.

The respiratory system has many mechanisms to reduce the amount of toxins entering our body. The hairs in our nose trap dust and pollutants, which are expelled when we blow our nose. Specialized cells lining our respiratory tract produce mucus which traps inhaled bacteria and debris. Other cells have fine hair on their surface called cilia. These beat rhythmically towards the larynx, thus encouraging debris to travel towards the throat, where it can be coughed out or swallowed. The alveoli contain large amounts of scavenger cells called macrophages which eat up debris, and help to prevent bacterial infections in the lungs.

Those of us who live in the city become accustomed to smog and exhaust fumes as a part of life. If we are exposed to the same chemical each day, we can stop noticing its presence. For example, office workers are exposed to toxins from the photocopier; nail technicians are exposed to fumes from various solvents; and painters regularly inhale a host of chemicals.

The Skin

Our skin is much more than just a protective covering; it is actually our largest organ of elimination. If working optimally, we can excrete a significant amount of water soluble toxins through the skin. Sweat has a composition similar to urine, and is an important detoxification fluid. This is why exercise is so vital to good health. Any exercise that makes you huff and puff pumps blood around your body under high pressure. This is great for improving your circulation and bringing blood to your extremities. Toxins can then be brought to the skin's surface and eliminated as perspiration. Saunas and steam baths can achieve a similar purpose.

Skin conditions such as acne, eczema and psoriasis are extremely common. Conventional medicine treats these as if something is wrong with the skin itself; when in reality they are usually manifestations of internal toxicity. If the other organs of elimination are over burdened or not functioning optimally, the skin will have the task of riding the body of excess toxins. You should find that your skin clears up well on our detoxification regime. However, when beginning any detox program, a temporary flare up of skin conditions is common, as a greater amount of toxins are eliminated.

Chapter Three

THE EFFECTS TOXINS HAVE ON OUR BODY

How Do Toxins Enter Our Bodies?

As we have mentioned, the average person is exposed to a great number of toxic substances nearly every moment of the day. These either come from the outside world, such as in our air and water, (exogenous), or they are generated within our own bodies through metabolism and the inadequate digestion of food (endotoxins).

Ways In Which Our Bodies Are Exposed To Toxins

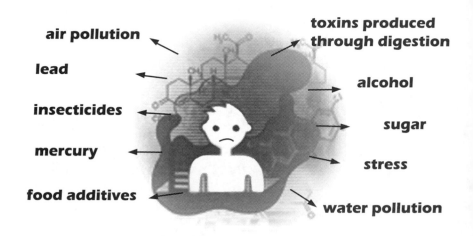

Air and water pollution
Cigarettes
Clothing
Building materials and furnishings
Food additives and contaminants (bacteria, mould, viruses)
Medications
Gut derived toxins (endotoxins)
Radiation
Cosmetics and toiletries
Household cleaners
Alcohol
Insecticides and pesticides in food
Heavy metals in the environment, foods and through occupational exposure
Stress
Excess sugar in the diet
Hydrogenated vegetable oils in the diet

What Are The Symptoms Of Being Overloaded With Toxins?

The symptoms of toxicity can be categorised into body systems. It will never be the case that toxins are only affecting one of your body systems; all systems are integrated. However, by looking at your symptoms you can check to see which parts of your body are burdened the most.

DIGESTIVE SYSTEM AND LIVER

- Abdominal bloating
- Nausea
- Coated tongue
- Bad breath (halitosis)
- Indigestion/heartburn
- Gas (burping or flatulence)
- Constipation or diarrhoea
- Body odour
- Overheating
- Irritable bowel syndrome
- Underweight or overweight

THE SKIN

- Rashes (eczema/dermatitis/hives)
- Acne and other blemishes
- Psoriasis
- Brown spots (liver spots)
- Clogged pores
- Excessive perspiration
- Dark circles under the eyes
- Puffiness under the eyes
- Red or itchy eyes

THE LYMPHATIC AND IMMUNE SYSTEMS

- Fluid retention/bloating
- Frequent infections
- Vasculitis
- Painful, swollen lymph nodes
- Allergies
- Autoimmune disease
- Fatigue
- Cellulite

THE MUSCULAR/SKELETAL SYSTEM

- Sore joints/arthritis
- Muscle aches & pains (fibromyalgia)
- Frequent headaches
- Tense muscles

THE URINARY SYSTEM

- Fluid retention
- Darkly coloured urine
- Strong smelling urine
- Frequent urinary tract infections (cystitis)

THE RESPIRATORY SYSTEM

- Chronic cough
- Wheezing
- Excess mucus/catarrh/post nasal drip
- Hayfever
- Sinusitis

THE NERVOUS SYSTEM

- Insomnia
- ADHD (Attention Deficit Hyperactivity Disorder)

- Mental fogginess
- Poor concentration
- Excessive sleepiness
- Muscle twitches
- Mild depression or anxiety
- Changeable moods

THE ENDOCRINE/HORMONAL SYSTEM

- Fluctuating blood sugar level (hypoglycemia)
- Sugar/carbohydrate cravings
- Overweight
- Excessive sweating and night sweats
- Unexplained infertility

Chapter Four

TOXINS IN OUR ENVIRONMENT

What Are Some Toxins That Can Impair Our Health and Where Are They Found?

As mentioned earlier, toxins can either come from outside our body, or be generated within our body. First we will examine some of the toxins in the outside world.

Air Pollution

This may be classified as outdoor air pollution or indoor air pollution. The major sources of outdoor air pollution are industry and motor vehicle emissions. Indoor air pollution originates mainly from the out gassing of chemicals from carpets, furniture, electrical equipment and household chemicals. Here are some major chemicals present in the air, and how they can affect our health:

- **Carbon Monoxide:**

Carbon monoxide is a colourless, odourless, and tasteless gas, which is highly poisonous. It is produced by the incomplete burning of natural gas, liquefied petroleum gas, wood, charcoal, coal, oil, gasoline and kerosene.

Common sources of carbon monoxide are motor vehicles, tobacco smoke, un-vented kerosene and gas heaters, gas stoves and gas water heaters, wood fireplaces and back-drafting from furnaces.

How Can Carbon Monoxide Affect Our Health?

Exposure to low levels of carbon monoxide can cause fatigue, chest pain, sweating, flu-like symptoms, memory loss, skin lesions and shortness of breath. Long term exposure may eventually lead to heart disease and damage to the nervous system. Carbon monoxide poisoning can cause death.

In pregnant women, carbon monoxide may cause miscarriage or increase the risk of damage to a developing foetus; it could also promote babies with low birth weights and nervous system damage.

- **Nitrogen Oxides:**

Nitrogen oxides are a group of gases that are made of nitrogen and oxygen. The two most common ones are nitric oxide and nitrogen dioxide.

Nitrogen oxides are mainly released into the air from motor vehicle exhaust, and the burning of oil, coal and natural gas, particularly from electric power plants. Cigarettes produce small amounts. Other processes that release nitrogen oxides are welding, electroplating, engraving, and dynamite blasting.

When they are combined with volatile organic compounds (carbon containing compounds), nitrogen oxides form ozone, or smog. Nitric oxide is used to bleach rayon. Nitrogen dioxide is used to produce rocket fuels, explosives and is sometimes used to bleach flour.

How Can Nitrogen Oxides Affect Our Health?

Long-term exposure to nitrogen oxides in smog may produce serious respiratory problems such as damage to lung tissue and reduction in lung function. Exposure may also irritate the eyes, nose, throat, and lungs. It can cause coughing, shortness of breath, nausea and fatigue.

Exposure to high industrial levels of nitrogen oxides can cause collapse, rapid burning and swelling of tissues in the throat and upper respiratory tract, difficult breathing and death if exposed to high enough quantities.

• Benzene:

This is a colourless liquid with a sweet odour, and is a kind of volatile organic compound. Benzene is produced from volcanoes and forest fires, and is a natural component of crude oil, gasoline, and cigarette smoke.

Benzene is used to produce other chemicals that are needed to make plastics, resins, nylon, and other synthetic fibers. It is also used to make explosives, photographic and printing chemicals, dyes, lubricants, paint, detergents, rubber, glue, pesticides and drugs. It is sometimes used as a gasoline additive.

How Can Benzene Affect Our Health?

Benzene has been known to cause cancer, and for this reason, is classified as a carcinogen by the US National Toxicology Program. Long term exposure to high levels may cause leukemia.

Long-term exposure to benzene can reduce your number of red

blood cells, leading to anaemia. It may also produce excessive bleeding and affect the immune system, increasing the risk of infection. Short term exposure to high levels of benzene affects the nervous system, and can cause paralysis, dizziness, chest tightness, sleepiness, rapid heart rate and coma.

• Ozone:

Ozone is a gas that is found both at the earth's ground level, and in the earth's upper atmosphere, where it occurs naturally and protects the earth from the sun's ultraviolet rays.

The ozone that occurs at ground level is the major component of smog. It is formed when sunlight reacts with pollution from motor vehicles and industrial sources. This occurs to a greater degree in summer due to the effects of higher temperatures and the sun. Ozone can also be industrially manufactured, and used for purifying air and drinking water; treating industrial waste; to control mold and bacteria in cold storage and to age liquor and wood.

How Can Ozone Affect Our Health?

Chronic exposure to ozone may cause permanent damage to the lungs, particularly in children whose lungs are still developing. It can cause breathing difficulties, chest tightness and throat irritation, and aggravate lung diseases such as bronchitis and emphysema. Ozone can cause reproductive and genetic damage, and suppress the immune system. Breathing ozone may cause headache, upset stomach, fatigue, vomiting and congestion.

• Sulfur Dioxide:

Sulfur dioxide is a colourless gas with a smell similar to a just-struck match. It is formed when fuel containing sulfur, such as oil and coal is burned. Most sulfur dioxide in the air comes from electric power plants. Other sources include cement manufacturing, petroleum refineries, copper smelting, paper pulp manufacturing and metal processing. Large ships, trains and some diesel equipment burn high sulfur fuel.

Sulfur dioxide concentrations in the atmosphere are highest in summer, when the sun and high temperatures react with pollution to form smog.

In addition, sulfur dioxide is used as a food preservative for some fruits (especially dried) and vegetables; for bleaching flour, textile fabrics and wool; as a disinfectant and for making other chemicals. It is also used in metal mining and refining, water treatment, and food processing.

How Can Sulfur Dioxide Affect Our Health?

Many people with asthma are sensitive to sulfur dioxide, and find that eating dried fruit containing preservatives, or being active outdoors aggravates their asthma. Sulfur dioxide in the air can react with other chemicals to form tiny sulfate particles; these can gather in the lungs and cause difficulty breathing, irritate the nose, throat and lungs and cause coughing.

Long-term chronic exposure to sulfur dioxide can cause chronic bronchitis and emphysema; it may also aggravate existing heart disease. Long term industrial exposure may impair fertility in men and women.

• Formaldehyde:

This is a colourless, pungent-smelling gas and a common source of indoor air pollution. It is a kind of volatile organic compound. Formaldehyde is used extensively by industry to manufacture building materials and numerous household products. It is also a by-product of combustion. Formaldehyde in the home can come from building materials, smoking, gas stoves, nail polish, new carpets, glues, foam insulation, paints and varnishes. It is used to add permanent-press qualities to clothing and draperies. Substantial amounts of formaldehyde can be released from new cars; especially those that have been sitting in the sun all day. The most significant source of formaldehyde in the home is pressed wood products made using adhesives that contain urea-formaldehyde resins. Such products include particleboard, hardwood, plywood paneling and medium density fiberboard.

Formaldehyde emissions usually decline as the product ages; therefore new houses can emit fairly high levels. High temperatures and humidity increase emissions.

How Can Formaldehyde Affect Our Health?

Formaldehyde can cause watery eyes, burning sensations in the eyes and throat, nausea, and breathing difficulties. High levels can trigger asthma attacks in asthmatics. Studies have shown that formaldehyde can cause cancer in animals. According to the 10th Report on Carcinogens, formaldehyde is "reasonably anticipated to be a carcinogen."

Low level exposure to formaldehyde may cause eye, nose, and throat irritation such as wheezing and coughing; skin rashes; fatigue and severe allergic reactions.

Fresh or Polluted Air?

Using air fresheners in your home can significantly increase the level of indoor air pollution. Air fresheners that plug into a power point release fragrance molecules such as pinene and limonene into the air. Studies have shown that when these molecules mix with ozone in the air, formaldehyde related compounds are formed, and can be present in concentrations of 50 micrograms in each cubic metre of air. This is close to the EPA's outdoor particle limit. When combined with formaldehyde emitting from furniture and other household chemicals, you could be breathing in quite a toxic cocktail. It's cheaper and healthier to eliminate the source of the odour, rather than trying to mask it. Ref. 3.

Water Pollution

Drinking eight to ten glasses of water each day is essential to maintaining good health. But just how pure is the water that comes out of our taps, and should we be drinking it? Approximately 60 000 tonnes of fifty different chemicals are used each year to treat the Australian water supply. Ref. 4. The main problems with the water supply are chlorine and its by-products, lead, bacteria, nitrates and organic compounds.

Chlorine is added to drinking water to control bacterial levels. Studies have shown that chlorinated water can act as a skin irritant, and may be associated with eczema. Chlorinated water may generate free radicals in the body, and can destroy polyunsaturated fatty acids and vitamin E in the body. Chlorine in the water destroys much of our beneficial intestinal flora, making us more susceptible to digestive upsets.

When chlorine mixes with organic compounds in the water (leaves, dirt), it forms what are called trihalomethanes. Chloroform is one of these chemicals. These chemicals are known to be carcinogenic, and they are stored in the fatty tissues of our body.

Lead can leach into the water supplies from solder and/or brass fittings in the hundreds of kilometers of underground pipes. Water standards in Australia state that lead levels cannot be above 50 parts per billion. Some Australian studies have shown lead levels of 12 to 300 times the safe limit. Ref. 5. Lead can cause mutations in foetuses, and can damage the nervous system; affecting learning and behaviour.

Bacteria can live and multiply in pipelines; feeding on slime which builds up over time. Bacteria levels may be acceptably low at storage sites, but increase substantially by the time our water reaches the tap. Some bacteria have developed a resistance to chlorine, and are not killed by it. Certain parasites such as giardia and cryptosporidium can occasionally turn up in the water supply also.

Nitrates that enter the water supply usually originate from pesticides that have contaminated ground water.

While looking for pesticide residues in tap water, researchers around the world have identified pharmaceutical drugs in the water supply. Drugs identified include painkillers, cholesterol lowering drugs, antibiotics, chemotherapy drugs, hormone residues from the contraceptive pill and HRT, anti-seizure medications and beta-blockers. It is quite a cocktail that comes out of our taps!

Cigarettes

Smoking cigarettes is willingly polluting your body with toxins. This habit will greatly increase the amount of free radical damage occurring in your body; increasing your chances of cancer, heart disease, and aging you more quickly.

According to the US Department of Health, here are 11 of the most toxic chemicals found in cigarette smoke:

- **Acetone** – This is a flammable, colourless liquid used as a solvent.

- **Ammonia** – Is a colourless, pungent gas. Ammonia enables you to   absorb more nicotine from the cigarette.

- **Arsenic** – Is a silvery-white metallic element. It is a poison used to make insecticides.

- **Benzene** – This is a flammable liquid obtained from coal tar and used as a solvent. Benzene is used to make many chemicals, from pesticides to detergent.

- **Benzoapyrene** – Is a yellow crystalline hydrocarbon found in coal tar. It is carcinogenic.

- **Butane** – This is a hydrocarbon used as a fuel. It is highly flammable and a key ingredient in gasoline.

- **Cadmium** – Is a metallic chemical element used in alloys. This metal accumulates in the body and can damage the liver, kidneys and brain.

- **Formaldehyde** – This is a colourless pungent gas used in solution as a disinfectan and preservative. It may damage the lungs, skin and digestive system, and may cause cancer. It is used by embalmers to preserve dead bodies.

- **Lead** – Is a bluish-gray toxic heavy metal. Lead poisoning can stunt growth and damage the brain.

- **Propylene Glycol** – This is a sweet hygroscopic (water attracting) viscous liquid used as antifreeze and as a solvent in brake fluid. It is used to keep tobacco from drying out and may aid in the delivery of nicotine to the brain.

- **Turpentine** – Is a colourless volatile oil. Turpentine is very toxic and is commonly used as a paint thinner.

Alcohol

When consumed in small amounts, alcohol is harmless, and can even benefit the body. Red wine is high in antioxidants, and all alcohol has a relaxing effect on the nervous system. However moderate to heavy drinking can create problems. It is estimated that one in six men and one in 12 women drink alcohol in quantities that may be damaging their health. Ref. 6.
Many people turn to alcohol at the end of a stressful day, as a way to wind down. However, some people become dependant on it, and come to need it daily just to feel okay. Regularly drinking more than 2 alcoholic drinks per day for women, and more than four for men, can create health problems. Binge drinking is even more harmful; this is where more than four drinks are consumed in a day.
When alcohol enters our body it is considered toxic, and must be broken down straight away. As alcohol is processed by the liver, other vital liver functions such as fat burning and detoxification will be put on hold. Therefore, you will find that losing weight becomes more difficult if you regularly consume alcohol.
Alcohol excess can affect our health in an acute or chronic way. Acute consequences can be the result of poor judgment and coordination, leading to motor vehicle accidents, drowning, sexual promiscuity, etcetera.

Chronic consequences can include the development of a fatty liver, and eventually cirrhosis of the liver; emotional problems such as depression; death of brain cells; an increased risk of certain cancers, such as breast cancer; and irritation to the digestive and urinary tract. Most cases of interstitial cystitis are aggravated by alcohol.

Caffeine

How well would you function if you were deprived of all caffeine for a day? Many of us wouldn't want to even consider this possibility. Consumed in small quantities, caffeine can help to make us more alert and improve our concentration. Coffee has some benefits; it contains the antioxidant chlorogenic acid, and the mineral magnesium. However, more than four cups of coffee a day can affect some people adversely.

Research from Duke University in the USA has shown that people who regularly consume more than 400mg of caffeine per day (roughly four cups of coffee), produce higher levels of stress hormones than those who consume less. Caffeine increases our heart rate and blood pressure. Excess consumption has been linked with cardiovascular disease and fibrocystic breast disease. Coffee may aggravate heartburn and ulcers because it increases the secretion of hydrochloric acid by the stomach. The more caffeine you consume, the more calcium you will lose in your urine.

A major problem with coffee is the high amount of pesticide residues it may contain. It is usually grown in Third World countries where toxic pesticides that have been banned in Western nations decades ago are still used. Organic coffee is readily available in most supermarkets and health food stores, and it may be a wiser option. Be careful if you drink decaffeinated coffee, that the caffeine has not been removed using toxic solvents. Choose coffee that has been water decaffeinated instead.

Coffee is the richest source of caffeine, but don't forget to think about other sources such as tea, cola soft drinks, energy drinks, guarana and chocolate.

Here is the approximate caffeine content of some foods:

- 1 cup instant coffee 60mg
- 1 cup espresso coffee 100mg
- 1 cup filter coffee 150mg
- 1 cup tea 50mg
- 1 can cola 35-46mg
- 50g bar dark chocolate 30mg
- 50g milk chocolate 15mg
- 250ml chocolate milk 8mg
- 1 can energy drink 80mg

Pesticides

A pesticide is any chemical that is used to control a pest. The pest may be an insect, weed, rodent, fungus, bacteria, fish or other bothersome organism. Currently, the application of chemicals is considered the most effective method for maximising crop yields. According to the CSIRO, world sales of agrichemicals (insecticides, fungicides, miticides, herbicides, acaricides) and plant growth regulators exceed $20 billion a year.

Pesticides can be classified into various groups. Here are some of the most common ones, and where they are likely to be used:

ORGANOPHOSPHATE INSECTICIDES

Acephane

Chlorpyrifos

Diazinon

These chemicals are typically found in lawn and garden sprays, household insect sprays, animal flea and tick collars and similar products, and agricultural sprays.

ORGANOCHLORINE INSECTICIDES

Endosulfan

Endosulfan is used to control insects on food and non-food crops and also as a wood preservative. It has oestrogen mimicking effects in the body.

SYNTHETIC PYRETHROID INSECTICIDES
Cyfluthrin
Cypermethrin
Deltamethrin
Permethrin
These chemicals are typically found in household and outdoor insecticides; also in termite control products.

INSECTICIDE/MITICIDE
Carbaryl
This chemical is used to control moths, mosquitos, beetles, ticks, cockroaches and ants. Carbaryl containing products are used on vegetables, fruits, lawns, ornamental plants and building foundations.

FUNGICIDES
Benomyl
Carbenadazim
Dithiocarbamates
Iprodione
Phosphoric acid
These chemicals may be used as a pre-harvest systemic fungicide, and as a post harvest dip or dust. They combat a wide range of fungal diseases in vegetable crops, soft fruit, mushrooms, nuts, ornamentals, tomatoes, lettuce and turf.

HERBICIDES
Glyphosate
Oryzalin
Oxyfluorfen
Pendimethalin
These chemicals kill weeds, and are found in products used to treat crops, forests, bodies of water, roadsides and lawns.

How Can Pesticides Affect Our Health?

The long- term effects of pesticide exposure are not clear. As a general rule, short- term high dose exposure may result in headaches, flu-like symptoms, nausea and irritability. Long-term exposure may harm the nervous system, cause hormonal imbalances and increase the risk of cancer. The extent to which pesticides affect you is largely dependant on your current state of health, the degree of your exposure, your age and genetic susceptibility, and your total body chemical burden. The foetus, infants and young children are most at risk of pesticide toxicity. Many pesticides are considered **endocrine disrupters.** This means that the chemicals may:

- Mimic a natural hormone; fooling the body into responding as if it were a hormone.
- Block the effects of a hormone.
- Directly stimulate or inhibit the endocrine (hormonal) system.

It is usually the sex hormones that are disrupted by pesticides. A well known example is the pesticide DDT, (and its metabolite DDE), which have potent anti-androgenic activity; meaning they block the effects of male hormones, or have a de-masculinizing action. Endosulfan is a relative of DDT, and has oestrogenic properties. Atrazine is a weed killer with broad hormonal activity. The well known book *Our Stolen Future* by Theo Colborn, Dianne Dumanoski and John Peterson Myers discus ses how hormone-like chemicals are lowering sperm counts in men, promoting early (precocious) puberty in children and increasing the rate of reproductive cancers.

What Can I Do To Minimize My Exposure To Pesticides?

When it comes to pesticides, prevention is better than cure. It can be quite hard for our bodies to get rid of pesticides, as many of them are fat soluble, and tend to accumulate in our fatty tissues and liver. Also, many pesticides are very long acting; some take approximately 40 years to finally breakdown.

The Environmental Working Group (EWG) is a US non-profit organization dedicated to protecting human health and the environment. According to their investigations, some fruits and vegetables contain much higher pesticide residues, and contain a greater variety of pesticides than others.

Based on the work of the EWG, these are the 12 most contaminated fruits and vegetables:

- Apples
- Capsicum
- Celery
- Cherries
- Grapes
- Nectarines
- Peaches
- Pears
- Potatoes
- Raspberries
- Spinach
- Strawberries

These are the 12 least contaminated fruits and vegetables:

- Asparagus
- Avocados
- Bananas
- Broccoli
- Cauliflower
- Corn on the cob
- Kiwi fruit
- Mangoes
- Onions

- Papaya
- Pineapple
- Peas

If you can buy organic fruits and vegetables, it may be worth it, particularly for those foods on the 12 most contaminated list. Also, try to vary the foods you eat as much as possible; avoid eating too much of any one fruit or vegetable. Wash fresh fruit and vegetables well before consuming, and some may be best peeled.

Toxins In Our Homes

Have you ever thought about just how many different chemicals you come into contact with in your own home; and how these chemicals may be affecting your health? Here we will look at some of the most common sources of chemical toxins in the home.

Cosmetics and Personal Care Products

Showering and grooming each morning usually involves the use of soap, shampoo, conditioner, deodorant, shaving cream, perfume or aftershave, hairspray, toothpaste; and that is before women apply any makeup. Our skin is highly permeable, allowing many toxic chemicals to enter our bloodstream.

Here are some of the nastiest ingredients commonly found in cosmetics, and the ones you are best off avoiding:

• **Phthalates** - These are a group of chemicals used to soften and increase the flexibility of plastic and vinyl. Phthalates are used in products including perfume, hair spray, shampoo, soap, nail polish, and skin moisturizers. They are also used in flexible plastic and vinyl toys, vinyl flooring, wallpaper, shower curtains, food packaging and plastic wrap. The most common phthalates used in cosmetics are dibutylphthalate (DBP), dimethylphthalate (DMP), and diethylphthalate (DEP). Their uses include plasticizers in nail polish (to make it less brittle, thus reduce cracking); in hair spray they help minimize stiffness, and allow a flexible film to form on the hair; and they are used as solvents and perfume fixatives in other products.

The human health effects of phthalates are not yet fully known, but are being continually studied. DEP is listed as a substance "reasonably anticipated to be a human carcinogen" in the 10th Report on Carcinogens. The National Toxicology Program concluded that high levels of DBP may adversely affect human reproduction or development. Phthalates in plastic thongs can be absorbed through the soles of the feet, and have been linked to erectile dysfunction in men.

- **Diethanolamine (DEA), Monoethanolamine (MEA) & Triethanolamine (TEA)** – These chemicals are often used in cosmetics to adjust the pH. They are also used to convert fatty acids to salts, which can be used as the basis of a cleanser. TEA can cause allergic reactions including eye problems, dryness of hair and skin, and could be toxic if absorbed into the body over a long period of time.

These chemicals are restricted in Europe due to known carcinogenic effects. According to Dr. Samuel Epstein (Professor of Environmental Health at the University of Illinois), "repeated skin applications . . . of DEA-based detergents resulted in a major increase in the incidence of liver and kidney cancer". Ref. 7.

- **Toluene** - Toluene is used as a solvent, and to make aviation gasoline, spray and wall paints, paint thinner, detergents, nail polish, medicine, dyes, explosives, spot removers, lacquers, adhesives, rubber, and antifreeze. Skin or eye contact with toluene can cause dryness, irritation and skin rashes. Inhalation irritates the upper respiratory tract. Exposure to low to moderate levels of toluene can cause confusion, light-headedness, dizziness, headache, nausea, fatigue, weakness, memory loss, coughing and wheezing. If you are pregnant, repeated exposure to toluene may increase the risk of damage to the foetus.

- **Formaldehyde** - Formaldehyde is a known carcinogen. It is commonly used as a preservative and solvent in personal care products. It may cause allergic, irritant and contact dermatitis, headaches and chronic fatigue. The vapour is extremely irritating to the mucous membranes, such as the eyes, nose and throat.

• **Mineral Oil** - This is a petroleum by-product that coats the skin like plastic, clogging the pores. It interferes with the skin's ability to eliminate toxins, promoting acne. Mineral oil is used in many products such as baby oil, moisturizers and personal lubricants. All mineral oil derivatives can be contaminated with PAHs (Polycyclic Aromatic Hydrocarbons), which are carcinogenic. Other names mineral oil can go by on ingredient labels are paraffin oil or paraffin wax and petrolatum. 95% of the chemicals used in perfumes and colognes come from petroleum.

• **Talc** - Studies have shown that regular use of talcum powder in the genital area is associated with a three-to-fourfold increase in the development of ovarian cancer.

• **Sodium Lauryl Sulfate** (SLS) & Ammonium Lauryl Sulfate (ALS) – These chemicals are used in 90% of products that foam, including shampoo, cleansers, car washes, floor cleaners and engine degreasers. SLS and ALS can irritate the eyes, and may even cause damage to the eyes of infants and children. Animals exposed to SLS and ALS experience eye damage, central nervous system depression, laboured breathing, diarrhoea and skin irritation.
Sodium Laureth Sulfate (SLES) and Ammonium Laureth Sulfate (ALES) are very similar compounds. When combined with other chemicals, they can form nitrosamines; potent carcinogens.

• **Hair Dyes** – These may contain a host of toxic chemicals, including heavy metals. Dark and red shades contain far more toxins than light shades. Their use may increase your chance of developing non-Hodgkin's lymphoma, leukaemia, multiple myeloma and Hodgkin's disease. Common ingredients in hair dyes include cadmium chloride, cobalt chloride, cupric chloride, lead acetate and silver nitrate. These are all highly irritating to the mucous membranes and can cause burns and rashes. Arylamine is an ingredient in hair dye strongly linked to the development of bladder cancer. Ref. 8.

There are a number of cosmetics companies that produce products free of all or most of these chemicals; they include *Jurlique, Aveda, Miessence, Botanique, Nui, Weleda* and *Alchemy*.

Household Products

Cleaning products you use around your home can contain quite toxic ingredients. Here are some commonly used products:

• **All Purpose Cleaners** – These are usually a combination of detergents, grease cutting agents, solvents and disinfectants. Ammonia in these products can irritate the eyes and lungs and cause skin burns or rashes. Do not mix ammonia containing cleaners with bleach containing cleaners because a toxic chloramines gas will form. Ethylene glycol and monobutyl acetate can be absorbed through the skin and are toxic. Inhalation can produce dizziness. Sodium hyperchlorite in these products is corrosive to the skin and eyes; the fumes irritate the respiratory tract.

• **Glass and Window Cleaners** – These commonly contain ammonia or isopropanol, water and colour. Isopropanol can be irritating to the eyes, skin, nose and throat.

• **Bleach** – Liquid cleaning bleach contains approximately five percent hypochlorite solution. Chlorine fumes are highly irritating to the eyes and respiratory tract. Direct skin contact can cause dermatitis. Bleach should never be mixed with other cleaners.

• **Paint** – Typically paint is comprised of 2-25% pigment and 75-95% solvent. The solvents commonly used in paint include mineral spirits (naphtha), toluene, xylene and other petroleum derived solvents. Oil based paints and varnishes are particularly high in solvent content. These solvents are irritating to the mucous membranes, and fumes may produce nausea, dizziness, headaches and fatigue. Respiratory conditions such as asthma can be aggravated. Due to their toxin content, pregnant women should never be exposed to paint, unless it is a non-toxic paint. *BIO Products* makes human friendly paints, varnishes, waxes and associated products.

Chemicals in the Kitchen

Take a good look at the cookware you are using to cook your meals. The synthetic lining on non-stick cookware can emit harmful toxins.

Perfluorochemicals (PFCs) are some of the most harmful chemicals ever developed. They are used to prevent food sticking to pots and pans, but also repel stains on furniture and rugs and make the rain fall off coats; keeping you dry. They are also used in food wrap, sprays for shoes and leather, paint, floor wax and shampoo. Some major brands containing PFCs include Teflon, Scotchgard, Stainmaster and Gore-Tex. PFCs are comprised of chains of carbon atoms of varying lengths, to which fluorine atoms are strongly bonded. This means the chemicals are virtually indestructible, and some members of the PFC family never degrade.

PFOA and PTFE are types of perfluorochemicals, and are used in the manufacture of Teflon. They are released into the air when Teflon cookware is heated to high temperatures. If you use this kind of non-stick cookware, you will be breathing in toxin fumes, and they will enter your food. It is well known that if you keep a pet bird in the kitchen while heating a non-stick pan to high temperatures, the bird can die. These fumes are highly toxic to birds!

Perfluorochemicals have been found in the blood of people everywhere. Nine studies were published between 1972 and 1989 on levels of PFCs in humans. Scientists have detected PFOA in the majority of samples tested from nearly 3000 US residents, including blood samples from 598 children, 238 elderly Washington State residents, and approximately 2000 blood bank donors. Ref. 9.

PFOA is claimed to promote four types of tumours; testicular, breast, liver and prostate. PFOA also causes hypothyroidism in laboratory studies. The levels of PFOA in some people's bodies now appear to be in the range known to harm animals.

What you can do to minimize exposure to PFCs

Here are some tips:

- Do not use Teflon or other non-stick cookware in your home. Stainless steel is the healthiest cooking surface. To prevent food from sticking use a little water, olive oil or butter.

- When purchasing furniture or carpet, do not have them treated to be stain resistant. This will prevent these chemicals emitting into your home.

- Do not buy clothing that bears the Teflon label, or indicates it has been treated for water, dirt or stain repellency.

- Minimize the amount of packaged and fast food in your diet. Often these containers are coated with PFCs to prevent grease from soaking through the packaging. PFCs are used in containers such as hot chip boxes, pizza boxes and microwave popcorn bags.

- Do not buy personal care products that contain "fluoro" or "perfluoro" in the ingredients list. They are commonly found in nail polish, pressed powders, lotions and shaving cream.

Tips for reducing the chemical load in your home

- If a fragrance or colour free version of a toiletry or cleaning product exists, choose it instead of the regular.

- Avoid chemicals you don't need to use, for example:

  a) Fly spray: use a fly swat instead and make sure all your fly screens are intact.

  b) Oven cleaner: these usually contain quite harsh chemicals; therefore it may be better to make sure you don't spill any food in the oven in the first place, to avoid having to use these chemicals.

  c) Air fresheners: get rid of the source of the odour instead.

- Go without makeup or perfume on days you don't have to go out, or use less on those days.

- Use environmentally friendly cleaning products that are low in phosphates or bio-degradable.

- Use cosmetics and toiletries that state they are free of petrochemicals.

- Use natural products as cleaning agents.
  Here are some ideas:

1. All purpose cleaner: for every 2 heaped tablespoons of bicarbonate of soda use 1 tablespoon of white vinegar. Mix together well and store in an airtight container.

2. Dishwashing rinse aid: use white vinegar to prevent spotting and streaking.

3. Mildew on fabrics: Fungus can be killed by hanging the fabric outside in the hot sun, or outside on a frosty night.

4. Cleaning windows and mirrors: Mix ½ cup white vinegar with 1 litre of water. Cold black tea can also be used.

5. To clean floor tiles: use 1 tablespoon of white vinegar and the juice of 4 lemons in a bucket of hot water.

Pollutants in plastic wrap

Toxins from cling film wrapping used to cover cheese, meat, fish and packaged fruit and vegetables can migrate into food. The chemicals DEHA and vinylidene chloride are both carcinogens, and are found in such packaging. They are also endocrine disrupters, because they have hormone-mimicking effects. Foods that are high in fat, such as meat and cheese seem to absorb more of these chemicals.

Do not microwave food in any kind of plastic containers. Microwaving can drive plastic molecules from the container, into your food. If you use microwaves, it is preferable to heat food in glass or ceramic containers. Use a paper towel to cover the food, rather than plastic wrap. Polystyrene (styrofoam) transfers toxins into the hot liquid held within it. So avoid takeaway coffee in polystyrene containers; take the time to sit down and have a coffee in a mug, and avoid coffee shops that only serve coffee in these containers.

Sugar

A high intake of sugar can place a great deal of stress on the body. It takes very little digesting, produces a rapid rise in the blood sugar level, usually followed by a slump in blood sugar, and energy. Nancy Appleton, PhD is the author of the book *"Lick The*

Sugar Habit"; she has listed 124 ways in which sugar can damage our health. Some of these include suppressing the immune system, depleting the body of minerals, promoting high triglyceride levels and increasing the risk of fatty liver disease.

Researchers at the New York State University in Buffalo, USA studied which foods produced the greatest amounts of free radicals in the body. Sugar came out on top. Within two hours of eating 300 calories of sugar, the amount of free radicals in the body increased by 140%. 300 calories of sugar is roughly equal to a can of soft drink and some chocolate; a common part of a lot of people's diet.

Sugar makes us age more quickly. Glucose can stick itself onto proteins in our body; this is called glycosylation. Glycosylation of proteins means their structure has been changed, causing them to bind, or cross-link together. This can happen to collagen, meaning it will lose elasticity, causing wrinkles. That's something even the latest, most expensive anti-aging cream can't repair!

Sugar can also increase gut toxicity, by feeding bad bacteria and yeast in our gut. This will increase the amount of fermentation in your gut, leading to bloating, and more toxins leaking through into your bloodstream.

Refined/Hydrogenated Vegetable Oils

Refined vegetable oil and most margarines are highly processed, toxic additions to any diet. Most people are not aware of how vegetable oil is manufactured, or that butter is a much healthier alternative to margarine. Oils are extracted from seeds and nuts with the use of heat and/or chemical solvents; they are then degummed, refined, bleached, and deodorized. The resultant oil is colourless, odourless and tasteless.

The manufacture of cooking oil involves the following processes:

- The addition of NaOH (sodium hydroxide) to remove the alkali-soluble minor ingredients from the oil. The minor ingredients have health benefits, but diminish the shelf life of the oil; therefore they are discarded. Incidentally, NaOH is a corrosive chemical used to burn clogged sinks and drain pipes open.

- H3PO4 (phosphoric acid) is added to remove the acid-soluble minor ingredients. These also have health benefits, yet would lead to faster spoilage if left inside. H3PO4 is a corrosive acid used commercially to degrease windows.

- Bleaching clays are used to obtain greater shelf stability. The clays damage the molecules that give oil its colour. Colour absorbs light, and the light would lead to a faster deterioration of the oil. Bleaching makes the oil rancid, which gives it a bad odour and flavour.

- Consequently, the oil is then deodorized. This takes place at frying temperatures (220 to 245 degrees Celsius). The resultant oil is colourless, odourless and tasteless; and because it is made of vegetables, is promoted as healthy. How many fast food outlets have you seen with a big sign proclaiming "We use 100% vegetable oil for cooking"? Or "Our oil is 100% cholesterol free". Now you know that this makes the foods cooked in this oil far from healthy.

Here are some of the minor ingredients removed from the oil during manufacture because it is not profitable to leave them in:

- Antioxidants including vitamin E and carotenes.
- Lecithin; which emulsifies oil and makes it easier to digest.

- Phytosterols; which have cardiovascular and immune benefits.
- Chlorophyll; which has a blood purifying effect, and is high in magnesium.

If you purchase these oils, then use them at home for frying; the light, oxygen and heat further damage the oil. The Essential Fatty Acids once present in the oil are long gone. This means they offer no health benefits and can be harmful.

Which Oils Are Healthy?

When purchasing oil, it must state on the label that it is unrefined or cold pressed. Extra virgin olive oil is unrefined; it is cold pressed (extracted without the use of heat), and still contains the minor ingredients with health giving properties. You will notice that this oil is thicker and a darker colour. A good quality brand will be in a dark glass bottle; protecting it from the damaging effects of light. "Lite" olive oil is no lower in fat or calories than the original; it is lighter in colour because it has been refined. When using oil, it is best added to food once it has already been cooked. However, small amounts of olive oil, butter and unrefined coconut fat can be used for cooking, because they are fairly heat stable. Cold pressed flaxseed oil, macadamia oil or walnut oil can be used, but they must never be heated.

Margarine: the same oil, damaged further

In most cases margarine manufacture involves the hydrogenation, or partial hydrogenation of vegetable oil. The oil is treated with hydrogen gas at high temperatures; it is artificially saturated with hydrogen atoms. This makes the product harder and spreadable. Hydrogenation of vegetable oil alters the configuration of the fatty acids from the natural cis, to the trans form. **Trans fatty acids** are foreign to the body. The liver certainly doesn't know what to do with them. They have been linked to the development of fatty liver, raised LDL (bad) cholesterol, cardiovascular disease and cancer.

Food Additives

Food these days is not simple. It is not good enough for food to just taste good and be nutritious. It must be fun: fun to eat, fun to unwrap, pretty to look at, convenient to carry around and have a long shelf life. To achieve this, food manufacturers have included a growing number of artificial additives in foods. Currently more than 3 000 additives are used worldwide in food. The majority of these chemicals are synthetic and foreign to the body. The more chemicals we have in our diet, the greater the workload on the liver to metabolize them. This detracts the liver from other vital functions such as cleansing the bloodstream and fat burning. Of all the additives in use currently, these are possibly the most troublesome:

• **Flavour enhancers:** These include the additives 620-637. Monosodium glutamate (MSG) is in this family and is represented by the code 621. This group of chemicals is capable of causing allergic reactions, ranging from a mild rash to anaphylactic shock. Facial flushing and headaches are also common reactions. Flavour enhancers are commonly found in potato and corn chips, instant noodles, flavoured crackers, microwave meals and takeaway foods and sausages.

• **Aspartame:** The main brands of this artificial sweetener are NutraSweet and Equal. Aspartame is made of phenylalanine, aspartic acid and methanol (a kind of alcohol). In the body, methanol breaks down into formaldehyde (a cancer causing substance); formic acid (an acid found in the venom of bees and ants); and diketopiperazine (shown to cause brain tumours in animals). Aspartame is found in many diet foods such as soft drinks, diet yoghurt, diet jelly and sugar free chewing gum.

• **Sulfites:** These include sulfur dioxide, sodium sulfite, potassium bisulfite, metabisulfite and bisulfite. This group of additives may trigger asthma attacks in sensitive individuals. They are commonly found in dried fruit, and products containing dried fruit such as muesli bars and breakfast cereals; desiccated coconut;

cordial, wine and sausages.

• **Propionates:** These are common bread preservatives and include the numbers 280-283. Calcium propionate is the most widely known additive in this group, and is represented by 282. Propionates occur naturally in some foods, such as Swiss cheese; however, some individuals are sensitive to them, and the effects are dose related. Calcium propionate is added to inhibit the growth of mould, thereby extending the shelf life of bread. Reactions to these additives can range from migraine and headaches; gastro-intestinal symptoms including stomach aches, diarrhoea; bedwetting; eczema; nasal congestion (stuffy or runny nose); impairment of memory and concentration; racing heart; irritability, restlessness and difficulty sleeping.

• **Antioxidants:** A range of antioxidants are used in food manufacture; they range from 300, which happens to be vitamin C, to 321 which is BHT; a harmful antioxidant. We usually think of antioxidants as having health giving properties, but some antioxidants added to foods are synthetic chemicals that have harmful effects in the body. The two additives to avoid are BHA (Butylated hydroxyanisole) and BHT (Butylated hydroxytoluene); represented by 320 and 321 respectively. BHA and BHT are used to prevent rancidity in oils, and are commonly found in margarine, dairy blend, crackers, biscuits, croissants, potato crisps and muesli bars. They may be present in takeaway food cooked in margarine containing these antioxidants. Side effects linked to BHA and BHT include asthma, insomnia, depression, tiredness, learning difficulties and children's behaviour problems.

• **Colours:** Synthetic colourings may produce allergic reactions in some individuals, and have been linked to learning and behavioural problems in children. The most common offenders are tartrazine (102) and annatto (160b). Other synthetic colours to avoid include 107, 110, 122-129, 132, 133, 142, 151 and 155. Ref. 10.

Now we will take a look at some of the toxins that are generated within our own bodies:

Chapter Five

TOXINS GENERATED WITHIN THE BODY

Stress

Stress can have a measurable effect on our health. Whenever
we have a negative thought or experience a negative emotion, a
chemical is released that affects our physical well-being. A field of
research called psychoneuroimmunology (PNI) studies the effects
that thoughts and emotions have on our physical health. Fear,
anger and resentment have been referred to as toxic emotions, and
they can certainly create a toxic state in our bodies.
Our initial reaction to stress is the flight or fight response; our

heart beats rapidly, we start to perspire, our pupils dilate, and we feel a surge of adrenaline. If the stress continues, our body copes by producing cortisol and other stress hormones from the adrenal glands. Long-term stress is detrimental because cortisol has a number of biological effects. It can suppress the immune system; inhibit digestive secretions, producing symptoms of irritable bowel syndrome; raise the blood pressure; cause fluctuating blood sugar levels (hypoglycaemia); impair memory and concentration; worsen fibromyalgia; and raise insulin levels, promoting weight gain.

If stress continues beyond this point, the body enters a state of exhaustion. The immune system suffers further, and susceptibility to disease greatly increases.

To add insult to injury, most people do not cope with stress in a productive, self nourishing way. Typically people deal with their frustrations by smoking, drinking more alcohol, comfort eating sweets or binge eating, gambling, shopping to excess, etcetera.

It is very important to look after yourself emotionally as well as physically, otherwise, good eating habits can be abandoned as soon as a major stress is encountered.

Poor Digestion

Our digestive tract is a major entry point of toxins into our body. This is understandable when we consider that the average person consumes more than 25 tonnes of food over their lifetime! To avoid creating toxins internally, your digestion must be good.

As mentioned earlier, saliva contains digestive enzymes, particularly amylase, needed for carbohydrate digestion. All too often people eat in a hurried manner, when stressed, or while their mind is engaged elsewhere, such as the television. This is a bad start. In the stomach hydrochloric acid and enzymes are secreted in order to digest protein. Stress inhibits all enzyme secretion and our production of hydrochloric acid declines as we get older. So many people routinely take antacids and other stomach acid blockers. These people will not be digesting protein adequately, and may experience abdominal bloating, reflux and burping.

In the small intestine bile from the liver; pancreatic juices and enzymes secreted by the intestinal lining act to digest food. Once again, stress and nutritional deficiencies can impair enzyme production. This can give you abdominal bloating, flatulence and abdominal cramps. Most absorption of nutrients occurs in the small intestine, so its lining must be healthy for adequate absorption to occur.

If there has been a lack of digestive enzymes, partially digested food reaches the large intestine and can putrefy and ferment. The problem is compounded if there is a lack of fibre and water in the diet. If you are constipated, or do not have a bowel movement each day, toxins inside your intestines are in contact with the intestinal wall for longer than desirable. This can increase the risk of bowel cancer. It also means that toxins will be absorbed through the bowel wall into your body; polluting your entire body.

Dysbiosis: Too many bad bugs

Another scenario that increases gut toxicity is the overgrowth of harmful gut flora, called dysbiosis. It is estimated that more than 500 species of bacteria are present in the human gut in concentrations of between 100 billion to 1 trillion microbes per gram. This adds up to about 95% of the total number of cells in the human body. Ref. 11. Ref. 12.

The good bacteria in the stomach and intestines can become unbalanced, making us vulnerable to the overgrowth of yeast, fungi, parasites and harmful bacteria. Poorly digested food, a high sugar diet and medication such as antibiotics alter the intestinal pH, and kill beneficial bacteria. This creates a perfect environment for dysbiosis. Candida overgrowth is a common manifestation of dysbiosis. Each of us have small amounts of Candida growing in our digestive tract; it is only when digestion is poor, and the immune system and liver are functioning poorly that Candida is allowed to flourish.

If you have bad digestion, your intestinal lining can become irritated and what is known as "leaky gut syndrome" can develop. This is discussed in greater detail on page 74. In susceptible individuals, incompletely digested food particles can seep into the bloodstream, challenge the immune system and lead to food allergies and intolerances. They can also interact with the immune system to form circulating immune complexes. These complexes can create inflammation, arthritis, fibromyalgia and autoimmune conditions such as Hashimoto's thyroiditis.

Food Allergies or Intolerances

Any food we are allergic or intolerant to acts like a poison in our body. There is a lot of truth to the saying "One man's bread is another man's poison". Only approximately 5% of people are born with an allergy. In the majority of cases food allergies and intolerances develop over time; so a food you once tolerated well in the past may be making you ill today.

If our digestion is poor, we are stressed, have nutritional deficiencies or take certain medications, we may develop what is known as "leaky gut syndrome". This is where the intestinal lining becomes more permeable than it should be, allowing toxins to gain entry into our bloodstream. This will also allow partially, incompletely digested food molecules to enter the bloodstream. This challenges the immune system, and over time we may develop an intolerance or allergy to a particular food. Very often the foods we are intolerant or allergic to are the foods we crave. The most common culprits are dairy products, wheat, eggs, soy, tomatoes and oranges.

Food allergies and intolerances can produce far ranging symptoms; some of the most common ones are:

- Fluid retention
- Abdominal bloating
- Irritable bowel syndrome
- Skin rashes such as eczema, psoriasis & acne rosacea
- Weight gain
- Headaches
- Mood changes
- Fatigue
- Foggy brain
- Cravings for sugar, bread & other carbohydrates
- Flu-like symptoms
- Joint or muscle aches
- Mouth ulcers

- Recurrent bladder infections or interstitial cystitis
- ADHD

Eating foods you are allergic or intolerant to can create a lot of inflammation in your body, weakening your immune system. Also, if you are allergic or intolerant to foods you consume, your body will try to dilute them; to minimize their harmful effects. This congests your lymphatic system and leaves you looking bloated and puffy.

Hidden Infections

Hidden infections in the body place a major stress on the immune system and detox pathways. You may have an ongoing infection that you can't get rid of, or find you get repeated infections. Repeated courses of antibiotics act to further weaken your immune system and disrupt your digestion.

You may not realize you have an infection; it may be hidden, or subclinical. Perhaps the only symptoms you suffer are occasional bouts of fatigue, aches and pains, headaches, intermittent fevers and night sweats. The infection could be viral, bacterial, fungal or parasitic. Common sites of infections are the teeth, gums, sinuses, the nails, ears, lymph glands, bones or intestines. If you eat a lot of sugar and processed foods you will be feeding these organisms and promoting their growth. Unfortunately some micro-organisms are resistant to antibiotics, or are in a location with poor blood supply, where the antibiotics cannot reach.

Bacteria can release exotoxins and endotoxins, while yeast and fungi release mycotoxins into your body. These substances can give you a hang over type feeling, making you feel drained of energy, groggy on waking and feel achy and bloated.

There is a blood test you can have to check your serum globulin levels. A normal range for globulin is 25-35g/L. If your globulin level is raised, it may indicate your immune system is fighting an infection, or that there is another source of inflammation in your body, such as autoimmune disease. CT scans, MRIs and full body scans are other diagnostic techniques that can detect hidden infected cysts or pockets of pus.

Chapter Six

SIMPLE WAYS TO DETOX YOUR BODY

Now we will look at the best ways to support the elimination of toxins by your body, to reclaim your health and energy. Because the food we eat is a major entry point of toxins into our body, we will naturally start in the digestive tract.

1. Ensure Healthy Bowel Function

Every day you make choices about which foods you eat. Prevention is better than cure, and you can greatly reduce the toxin load on your body by choosing healthier foods. Try to eat food as close to its natural state as possible, rather than foods that have been through many different factory processes to arrive at the final product. Organic food is preferable, but not essential for good health. Do the best you can with what you have available.

The way we digest our food has a great bearing on the amount of endotoxins generated within our digestive tract, and then absorbed into our body. Here then are some common sense tips to ensure you digest your food as well as possible:

- Eat slowly and chew well. Do not bolt your food down. If you do not chew your food thoroughly, bacteria, yeast and fungi in your digestive tract will feast on it. This can lead to fermentation, leaving you bloated and suffering with gas.

- Try to eat only when you are calm and relaxed. There are more nerve fibres surrounding our gut than are in our brain, so our digestion is hugely affected by our emotional state. Stress impairs the secretion of digestive enzymes. If you are having a particularly stressful day, week, month (or life), take a deep breath before you begin your meal to try and slow your mind down. This will not only help your digestion, it should also help to prevent you becoming overweight. If you eat while doing two other things at the same time, you are more likely to overeat and want to snack later.

- Include raw foods in your daily diet. Raw vegetables and fruit are high in beneficial enzymes that help us digest our food. These enzymes are destroyed by heat. If most of the food you eat is cooked, your own body must work harder to produce these enzymes.

- Don't overeat. Eat until you are comfortably satisfied. We live in a country of plenty; you can always go back for more food later if you feel hungry. This will be much easier to achieve if you have eaten slowly and mindfully.

- Avoid drinking large volumes of water while eating because it can dilute digestive juices. Do most of your drinking between meals.

- Include bitter foods in your diet. When we taste bitter foods, nerve endings on our tongue travel to our digestive organs and stimulate digestive secretions. Examples of bitter foods include radicchio lettuce, chicory, endive and bitter melon

Treat Leaky Gut Syndrome

Leaky gut syndrome is an extremely common condition which may be at the root of your health problems.

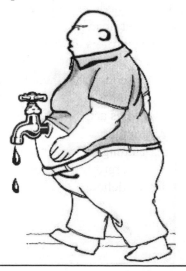

What is leaky gut syndrome?

The lining of our small intestine is designed to allow nutrients we have digested to be absorbed into our bloodstream. Many kinds of beneficial bacteria and yeasts live here, helping us to digest and absorb substances. A leaky gut occurs when the mucous lining of the gut has become irritated and inflamed, making it more porous than it should be. This allows undigested food molecules, bacteria, fungi, metals and toxic substances to gain entry into our bloodstream. These toxins flood our liver, and then spill into the bloodstream. If allowed to flourish, Candida will grow in the mucous membrane lining like a large tree where the roots cause cracks in the surrounding concrete. The roots of the Candida can worsen the leaks in the gut. If Candida is allowed to enter the bloodstream it can travel to various parts of the body and promote fungal infections; examples include tinea, thrush and jock itch. The immune system becomes overwhelmed by all of these toxins and reacts by producing antibodies and inflammatory chemicals. Leaky gut syndrome is strongly associated with several autoimmune diseases. Ref. 13 .

What causes leaky gut syndrome?

The following are all possible causes:
- Overuse of medications such as antibiotics, steroids and non-steroidal anti-inflammatory drugs, such as aspirin, ibuprofen and naproxen.
- Poor diet high in sugar, refined carbohydrates and processed foods (eg. Soft drinks, white bread, sweets).
- Stress.
- Food allergies and intolerances.
- High consumption of alcohol.
- Food poisoning and gastrointestinal infections.
- Candida overgrowth
- Nutritional deficiencies

What are the symptoms?

- Irritable bowel syndrome or indigestion
- Abdominal bloating and/or flatulence.
- Candida infections & other fungal infections such as thrush, tinea, jock itch.
- Allergies to foods, airborne substances or chemicals.
- Chronic fatigue and weakened immunity.
- Deficiencies of minerals, fat soluble vitamins and Essential Fatty Acids.
- Joint pain.
- Foggy head or clouded thinking.
- Autoimmune diseases such as rheumatoid arthritis, lupus, thyroid disease.

How to Overcome Leaky Gut Syndrome

- Remove excess Candida and other harmful yeast, fungi and bacteria. There are certain powerful herbs that act as natural anti parasitics, including Berberis, wormwood and thyme. You can read more about these herbs on page 77.

- Don't feed what you are trying to kill. Sugar feeds yeast in your gut, so your diet must be free of sugar and foods made of white flour. Reducing your general intake of grains can help, because they are all digested into sugar in your intestines.

- Follow a low reactive diet. This means avoid the foods that most commonly promote or aggravate a leaky gut. These include dairy products, gluten and possibly others.

- Strengthen your immune system. Killing off Candida and parasites is important, but if your immune system is weak they will be allowed to overgrow again.

- Avoid alcohol, and if possible minimize the use of non steroidal anti inflammatory drugs and antibiotics.

- Include chilies, raw garlic and onion in your diet, as they have antibacterial properties.

- You may require a digestive enzyme supplement to help you digest your food more thoroughly, and make you more comfortable after meals. A good one would contain the enzymes, amylase, protease, lipase and cellulase.

- Take a probiotic supplement containing beneficial bacteria such as lactobacillus acidophilus and bifidobacterium bifidum. Good bacteria in the gut can crowd out harmful organisms.

- Prebiotics are natural plant fibres that promote the growth of good bacteria in our gut; they are food for the good bacteria. An example of a prebiotic is FOS (fructooligosaccharides); this can be obtained in supplement form, but is also found in the vegetable Jerusalem artichoke.

The Benefits of Specific Anti-parasitic Herbs

BERBERIS
The common name for this herb is barberry; it has been used to treat diarrhoea in China and India since ancient times. The stem bark and root bark of berberis are used. The active ingredient of berberis is a bitter, yellow alkaloid called berberine. This substance increases the flow of bile from the liver; helping to cleanse the liver and improve digestion. Berberine has demonstrated antimicrobial activity against a variety of organisms such as bacteria, viruses, fungi, Candida, protozoans, helminthes

(worms), and Chlamydia. Ref. 14. It is effective in treating diarrhoea caused by E. coli infection. Ref. 15.

WORMWOOD

This herb, also known as Artemisia has traditionally been used to rid the body of intestinal worms and parasites. It also stimulates bile flow in the liver and promotes bowel regularity. New research has shown that wormwood may have anti-malarial effects. Ref. 16.

THYME

It is believed this herb comes from the Greek word thumus, which means courage. Thyme was once used to give soldiers courage and invigoration. In modern times it is recognized that thyme has powerful antibacterial, antiviral and antifungal effects. Ref. 17. Thymol is the powerful antiseptic found in thyme. It is an excellent treatment for many types of infections, and has even shown effectiveness against Helicobacter pylori infections. Ref. 18.

You can find these three most effective cleansing and antiseptic herbs in the Detox & Slim 1.2.3. formula. **For more information about these herbs please call our Health Advisory service on 02 4655 8855.**

OLIVE LEAF EXTRACT

Olive leaf is another powerful antimicrobial substance. The active ingredient is called oleuropein. This compound is produced by olive trees in order to make them resistant to insect and bacterial damage. In our gastrointestinal tract olive leaf has infection fighting properties. Olive leaf needs to be taken in a higher dose, therefore is best taken alone, or combined with small amounts of zinc and the herb Andrographis paniculata.

SOOTHING SLIPPERY ELM

Slippery elm is a small tree common to parts of North America. The botanical name of slippery elm is Ulmus rubra, and it is the inner bark which is made into a powder and used medicinally. The 'slippery' part of the name refers to the texture of the herb. The inner bark is high in mucilage content, which is responsible for its wonderful healing and soothing action. The mucilage is a complex mixture of polysaccharides that form a gelatinous fibre when combined with water. Slippery elm is said to have a 'demulcent' or 'emollient' action, which means it is a soothing substance. Therefore, slippery elm has the ability to soothe and heal skin and mucous membranes it comes into contact with.

Traditionally the powdered bark has been used by Native Americans as a poultice for wounds, especially boils and ulcers. It was also made into porridge and consumed to treat gastrointestinal inflammation; this being its main use today. Slippery elm is an excellent remedy for leaky gut syndrome, irritable bowel syndrome, and any inflamed states of the digestive tract. It has a normalising effect on the stool, thus is used for constipation and diarrhoea.

Slippery elm can now be conveniently purchased in capsule form, and an ideal dose would be two to three capsules, three times daily. **For more information about slippery elm please call our Health Advisory service on 02 4655 8855.**

Avoid Constipation

The average person eats three meals a day, and possibly snacks as well, which would ideally produce between one and three bowel motions each day. The longer the stool is left to remain in the colon, the greater the amount of toxins will be reabsorbed into the bloodstream. The longer the bowel wall remains in contact with toxins, the more time bacteria in the colon have to transform substances in the stool into a more toxic state.
Many people who get headaches find that they are more painful and frequent if they are constipated. Retaining the toxins we are supposed to excrete in bowel movements is one of the most common ways we pollute our own bodies. Toxins that seep through the bowel wall often end up in the tiny lymphatic vessels;

eventually clogging the entire lymphatic system with toxins. The more regular your bowel movements, the better able your body is at excreting toxins.

Tips for avoiding constipation

- Drink approximately two litres of pure water each day. This will soften the stool and enable it to be passed more easily.
- Be more active. Exercise stimulates peristalsis, or intestinal contractions.
- Eat a diet high in vegetables, fruit, nuts and seeds and legumes.
- When you wake, drink a cup of warm water with the juice of half a lemon. The lemon will stimulate the production of bile, which is the body's own laxative; and the warm water will relax the bowel muscles.
- A black cup of coffee in the morning can work well for nervous constipation by relaxing the nerves surrounding the gut. Conversely, too much tea can be constipating due to its tannin content.
- Answer the call of nature. When it's time to go it's time to go.
- Take a fibre supplement, which acts as a gentle, non habit forming bulk laxative. If you regularly get constipated, some fecal matter is likely to get trapped on the walls of your bowels, and get left behind when you do have bowel motions. These deposits can be perfect breeding grounds for bacteria, leading to infections. A good fibre supplement should be free of gluten and psyllium, which are irritating to some people. It should contain fibre from more gentle sources, such as rice and soy bran and pectin. This combination of fibre acts to sweep your colon like a broom, keeping it clear of toxic waste matter.

For more information about fibre supplements, please call the Health Advisory Service on 02 4655 8855.

2. Support Healthy Liver Function

The liver is the most important detoxification organ in your body. It is where all of the toxins that get into your body are processed. The better your liver functions, the better able you will be to remove toxins, rather than having them build up in your fatty tissues.

As mentioned earlier, detoxification in the liver occurs in two steps. Phase one enzymes bio-activate toxins, and phase two enzymes neutralize them. The end products of phase one reactions are usually even more harmful than the original compound. So if we do not obtain enough antioxidants in our diet, these reactive intermediate compounds can do a great deal of harm in our liver, and throughout our body.

The problem with living in today's world is that so many of the substances we are exposed to in daily life activate the phase one liver enzymes. Due to poor health and nutritional deficiencies, the phase two enzymes lag behind.

The following substances are capable of inducing Phase one P450 enzymes. This means they can make these enzymes much more active; and hence generate a lot more free radicals in the process. Common inducers of P450 enzymes include:

- Alcohol
- Acetate
- Dioxin
- Exhaust fumes
- Sulfonamides (a type of antibiotic)
- Paint fumes
- Organophosphate pesticides
- Carbon tetrachloride
- Steroid hormones
- Stress
- Obesity
- Chronic inflammation
- Nicotine

- Selective serotonin reuptake inhibitor antidepressants
- Caffeine

If you want to enhance the detoxification ability of your liver, and minimize your body's toxic load, first of all try to avoid the above substances as much as possible.

Here are some more practical tips for improving your liver's detox ability:

- **Follow a liver friendly diet.** Make sure you eat lots of vegetables, fruit, protein and adequate Essential Fatty Acids. Your day to day diet has the greatest impact on your liver health.

- **Increase the amount of raw food in your diet.** This means eating a raw vegetable salad each day. Many antioxidants, nutrients and phyto chemicals in fruit and vegetables are destroyed by heat. These beneficial chemicals are essential to mop up the free radicals created in phase one of detoxification. Raw foods are also high in enzymes, which will improve your digestion. This is why raw vegetable juices are so beneficial for the liver. You can read more about their benefits on page 94.

- **Eat foods that are high in natural organic sulphur.** These foods include eggs, cruciferous vegetables (eg. Cauliflower, broccoli, Brussels sprouts & cabbage) and vegetables in the onion family, such as onions, garlic, leek and shallots. Sulphur is needed by the liver to carry out phase two detoxification. Sulphur containing amino acids such as taurine and cysteine are necessary for the production of bile. It is important not to have sluggish bile flow, because this is a major exit route for toxins that the liver has broken down. Sulphur foods promote better bile flow. You can take an organic sulphur supplement in powder form called MSM.

- **Avoid trans fatty acids.** These are usually found in vegetable oils that have been processed with heat, as well as margarine. You will find these fats on food labels under the name hydrogenated, or partially hydrogenated vegetable oil. Trans fatty acids have an altered, un-natural shape. Fatty acids form our cell membranes so you do not want these fats making up your cells, because they will impair the cell's functions. Trans fats may promote the development of fatty liver.

- **Include "bifunctional modulators" in your diet.** These help you to achieve balanced detoxification. They are substances that modulate phase one enzyme activity, induce phase two activity, and minimize the free radical damage caused by reactive intermediates.

The following are examples of bifunctional modulators; try to include as much of them in your diet as possible:

- **Green tea**. Catechins are a group of antioxidants found in green tea. They are reputed to be 200 times more powerful an antioxidant than vitamin C. Catechins are capable of inducing phase two liver enzymes. Ref. 19. Polyphenols are another class of antioxidant found in green tea. Green tea also promotes healthy bowel function, so make sure you drink at least a cup a day.

- **Sesame seeds.** Sesamin is a component of sesame seeds, and it is a powerful hepatoprotectant; meaning it protects liver cells from toxic damage. It seems to especially protect the liver from the damaging effects of alcohol and carbon tetrachloride. Ref. 20. Sesamin is a powerful antioxidant, and reduces the breakdown of vitamin E in the body; helping to increase its concentration in the body.

- **Cruciferous vegetables.** This family of vegetables includes broccoli, cauliflower, cabbage and Brussels sprouts. These vegetables are the highest source of glucosinolates and isothiocyanates; substances that induce certain phase two enzymes. Glucosinolates are also found in mustard and horseradish, and give these foods their hot taste. Sulforaphane is one such substance found particularly in broccoli. It is one of the most powerful inducers of phase two enzymes known. Indole-3-carbinol is another beneficial substance in cruciferous vegetables; it is capable of beneficially altering oestrogen metabolism.

- **Watercress.** This herb is in the cruciferous vegetable family. It contains high levels of the isothiocyanate called phenylethyl isothiocyanate (PEITC). This chemical promotes the excretion of carcinogens in people, and inhibits chemically induced lung and colon cancer in rats. Watercress induces certain phase two liver enzymes, and may reduce the tendency to form fatty liver. Ref. 21.

- **Turmeric.** The active compound in turmeric is curcumin, and it has many antioxidant properties. Turmeric reduces the carcinogenic damage caused by cigarettes and reduces free radical damage to DNA. It increases glutathione production; the body's most powerful antioxidant. Ref. 22.

- **Silymarin**. This is the active component of the herb St Mary's Thistle. Silymarin is a hepatoprotectant, and increases the levels of glutathione in the body. Clinical trials have shown that a daily dose of 420mg is most beneficial.

- **Limonene.** This is a constituent of citrus fruits and caraway seeds. It is capable of blocking the harmful damage caused by many different carcinogens.

Other Nutrients That Support Liver Detoxification

If your diet is deficient in vitamins, minerals, protein or Essential Fatty Acids, you will have impaired detoxification.
The following are important for optimal detoxification to occur:

• Glycine
This is an amino acid necessary for bile production, and for phase two detoxification in the liver. When Kupffer cells of the liver engulf foreign substances, they can cause damage to liver cells. Glycine can minimize this damage. Ref. 23.

• Taurine

This is a sulphur containing amino acid that is essential for healthy bile production. It helps the liver to excrete toxins and cholesterol through the bile. Taurine is made from the amino acids methionine and cysteine, but humans have a limited ability to synthesize it. Therefore a taurine supplement can be very useful. Taurine can help to protect the liver against the damaging effects of alcohol, and reduce the tendency to form fatty liver. Ref. 24.

• Cysteine

This is a sulphur containing amino acid needed for the production of taurine. Cysteine is a precursor of glutathione, which is a powerful antioxidant. Cysteine helps to protect us from damage caused by alcohol and rancid fats.

• Methyl donors

These include the B vitamins; especially folic acid, as well as biotin and inositol. Methylation occurs in the liver, and is particularly important in detoxifying fat soluble chemicals and heavy metals.

A good liver tonic should contain the above nutrients as well as the herbs St Mary's Thistle and green tea. Please call our Health Advisory on 02 4655 8855 if you would like more information about liver tonics.

3. Keep your immune system strong

Your immune system is your greatest health asset, protecting you from an increasing number of new and exotic viruses, antibiotic resistant bacteria, fungi and parasites. The immune system is the protector of the body, and is itself worthy of protection and support, as it deals with the challenges of pathological "superbug" invaders.

Many people suffer with immune system degradation and inexplicable afflictions brought on by disease-causing micro-organisms. An increasing number of these micro-organisms have become resistant to the drugs we have relied upon for years and it has become vitally important to harness the antibiotic properties of the organic and yet powerful herbs and foods that we find in our natural environment.

A healthy and well balanced immune system will –
Reduce your risk of cancer
Reduce your risk of allergies
Reduce the occurrence of auto-immune diseases
Reduce the risk of degenerative diseases such as Alzheimer's dementia
Help you to fight off infections from bacteria, viruses and parasites
Improve your well being and energy levels

As we get older our immune system becomes more prone to malfunction, which leads to a greater risk of excess inflammation, auto-immune diseases, cancer and infections. It's worth investing some extra time and effort into strengthening your immune system. **Several factors can overload or weaken the immune system such as –**

- Toxic chemicals from cigarettes, pollution, plastics, insecticides and solvents, etc
- Excess sugar and refined carbohydrates in the diet, as if blood sugar levels rise we become more susceptible to infections
- Certain medications such as steroids, anti-inflammatory drugs and chemotherapy. The overuse of antibiotics in commercially produced meat encourages the growth of resistant bacteria called "superbugs"
- Stress especially if it is prolonged
- Sleep deprivation
- Liver dysfunction because the liver is the filter and

cleanser of the blood stream; those with a fatty liver are more susceptible to accumulate fat-soluble toxins in their liver and body

- Recurrent or chronic infections can get a foot hold in the body and release toxins that damage the immune system; these infections may be hidden and undiagnosed and manifest as chronic fatigue
- Exposure to unhealthy environments such as recycled air from jet liners, crowded rooms and buildings with poor ventilation or contaminated air conditioning systems (sick building syndrome)
- Deficiencies of antioxidants such as vitamin C, vitamin A (or betacarotene), vitamin E and the minerals selenium and zinc
- Food allergies such as intolerance to gluten, dairy products or artificial additives
- Lack of exercise and proper breathing, leading to poor oxygenation of tissues

If you think your immune system is not functioning well see your doctor for some tests. Useful and inexpensive tests for the immune system consist of –

A blood test to check –

- A full blood count to check the red and white blood cells
- An ESR (Erythrocyte Sedimentation Rate) – a high ESR is a marker of excess inflammation in the body
- The proteins called Immunoglobulins – if these proteins are elevated this is a sign of excess inflammation or infection
- Liver and kidney function
- A microscopy and culture of the urine

There are several practical strategies that you can use to support the healthy function of your immune system.

1. Raw juicing is a powerful way to boost your intake of antioxidants and phyto-chemicals to put out the fire of inflammation. Raw vegetables and fruits contain active enzymes, natural antibiotics and vitamins. Raw juicing is able to concentrate these invaluable substances in a form that is easily digested and absorbed.

A juice recipe to achieve this is-

½ cup chopped purple cabbage

1 large carrot

½ beetroot

1 orange (peel off the skin first, but leave the white pith as it contains bioflavonoids)

2 slices of red onion

1 clove garlic (optional)

1/4 cup chopped fennel

1 cm slice ginger root

2 red apples (you can use more if the taste is too strong)

Wash, chop and pass through the juicer and drink immediately.

2. Increase your intake of vitamin C as it is essential for the healthy function of white blood cells. Recommended doses are 1000 to 2000mg of vitamin C daily. Vitamin E has also been shown to enhance immune function.

3. Ensure that you are getting enough of the mineral selenium. It is best to take a selenium supplement containing the organic form of selenium, which is called selenomethionine. Selenium is vital for a healthy immune system and unfortunately is often deficient in Australian and New Zealand soils. Selenium is an anti-oxidant mineral that can reduce inflammation and auto-immune dysfunction. Selenium can reduce the incidence of infections from viruses and parasites and selenium has been dubbed "the viral birth control pill". This is due to its proven ability to reduce the capacity of viruses to replicate themselves. Selenium also has proven anti-cancer properties. The mineral zinc helps selenium to work more efficiently and can also reduce the incidence of infections and allergies.

4. Use natural antibiotics such as garlic, the herbs barberry, wormwood, thyme, horseradish root, ginger root, chili, turmeric, fenugreek and red onion; these things can be used in cooking, salads or raw juices. Foods high in organic sulphur compounds act as natural antiseptic cleansers and consist of vegetables from the cruciferous family such as broccoli, Brussels sprouts, cabbage, kale, bok choy and cauliflower.

Olive leaf extract has been used as a natural antibiotic for thousands of years. It is only over the last 30 years that scientific research has shown that its active ingredient oleuropein has healing properties and can inhibit the growth of bacteria, viruses, fungi and parasites that have the potential to cause infections. In 1995 the active components in olive leaves, elenolic acid and calcium elenolate were first isolated. This discovery provides society with a highly effective food supplement to act as a disease preventative. Olive leaf extract works to reduce the severity of colds, influenza and a broad range of other viruses, yeast, fungal and mould infestations, bacterial infections and parasites. If used in a high enough dosage olive leaf extract can help to expel worms from the intestines and is helpful for those with unhealthy micro-organisms in the gut. These results have been published in many different journals and are taken from the clinical experiences of practicing health professionals utilizing olive leaf extract for patients with infections and immune dysfunction. Research into olive leaf extract done in Hungary has shown such positive results against a broad range of infections that the Hungarian Government has adopted olive leaf extract as an official anti-infectious disease agent on its Medicare system. Olive leaf extract can be taken in capsule or liquid form.
In 1969 the research of Dr Renis working with the Upjohn Company proved that a compound of oleuropein from olive leaves could kill all viruses tested, including the herpes virus. The virucidal (virus killing) activity of oleuropein was due to

its interaction with the protein coat of the virus. In 1992 French biologists working at the Laboratoire de Pharmacognosie, Faculte de Pharmacie in Rennes France, found that all of the herpes viruses tested were inhibited or killed by olive leaf extract.

Other plants that exert antiseptic properties are tea tree and eucalyptus. If you suffer with recurrent respiratory infections such as sinusitis, pharyngitis and bronchitis, steam inhalations using 1 to 2 drops of tea tree oil or eucalyptus oil, can reduce the amount of unhealthy micro-organisms in the respiratory tract.

5. Dietary changes

It is important to have a diet that is abundant in antioxidants and vitamins. Generally speaking this means that you need to eat unprocessed foods found in their natural state and at least 6 to 8 servings of fresh fruits and vegetables daily. Everyone knows that it's important to eat vegetables that are green, orange and yellow in colour to provide vitamin K, chlorophyll, sulphur and the powerful antioxidants known as carotenoids.

It is just as important to consume regular amounts of red and purple coloured vegetables and fruits, as these contain plant chemicals known as anthocyanins. Anthocyanins are the pigments that give vegetables and fruits their deep purple and red colours and these pigments are vital for a healthy immune system. They are found in beetroot, purple cabbage, red onions, eggplant, purple sweet potatoes, red radish, red capsicums, purple asparagus, red basil, red chilies, berries, cherries, red grapes, plums, prunes, red apples, red pears, rhubarb and cranberries and tomatoes. Anthocyanins work very hard in your body acting as anti-inflammatory agents, antioxidants and even as natural antibiotics.

Scientists at Tufts University, Boston, studied the antioxidant power of various foods and found that blueberries were the most potent, with prunes, blackberries, raisins and strawberries close behind. There is considerable excitement about the potential of anthocyanins to reverse some of the degenerative changes in the brain caused by free radicals during the ageing process.

The antioxidant called lycopene is high in tomatoes, and pink coloured fruits such as guava, pink grapefruit and watermelon.

Lycopene reduces the incidence of various cancers such as cancer of the cervix, breast, lung and prostate gland. The body finds it easier to absorb and utilize lycopene from tomatoes if they are cooked (especially in a healthy oil) or from a tomato paste.

Here are some food suggestions to increase your intake of anthocyanins –

Use berries in smoothies – for slimmers add some whey protein powder which also has benefits for the immune system

Add berries to your breakfast cereals or porridge

Add pureed red vegetables to your soups

Use tomato paste in your stir fry or casseroles

Include red and purple coloured vegetables and fruits in your raw juices

Use shredded purple cabbage and red onions and red capsicums in your salads

Add egg plant thinly sliced to your stir fry

You can also roast these red vegetables in the oven – whole beetroots, purple sweet potatoes etc. – scrub them first, once cooked, slice, and mix with olive oil, balsamic vinegar, black pepper and other herbs as desired.

If you have frequent respiratory infections associated with a large amount of excess mucus and congestion try substituting dairy products with other milks such as coconut, unsweetened soy, almond, rice or oat milk. In some people this works wonders! Many people with recurrent infections and/or allergies are overweight and/or consume too much sugar in the form of refined carbohydrates. If the blood sugar levels are elevated, unhealthy micro-organisms tend to flourish and grow readily, as they are fed by the sugar. The worst sources of this excess sugar are candies, lollies, sweet cakes, biscuits, cookies, ice cream, soft drinks, cordials, refined flour breads and pastas. You can replace these high sugar foods with products made from unrefined flour and grains, or try replacing the grains with legumes (beans, peas, lentils). Low-carb-guilt-free varieties of chocolate bars are now available for those who love the taste of chocolate – isn't that everyone?

You can also replace sugar with the naturally sweet herb called Stevia, which does not raise blood sugar levels and is calorie free. Stevia is available in the form of liquid, tablets or powder and can be used to sweeten hot beverages and used in recipes for cakes and ice cream etc. For more ideas on how to use stevia, phone 02 4655 8855.

Healthy fats are also important for the immune system and can be found in oily fish (salmon, sardines, tuna, and mackerel), salmon oil, cold pressed olive oil and flaxseed oil, and raw nuts and seeds.

Our 2 week-detox program will cleanse the liver and reduce the work load of the immune system, enabling the immune system to strengthen. For those who wish to maintain a strong immune system we recommend the use of super foods, herbs and nutrients such as –

*   Barley leaf grass
*   Tenderstem
*   Beetroots
*   Carrots
*   Cabbage
*   Kelp
*   Spinach
*   Artichoke
*   Dandelion root
*   Gingko biloba
*   St Mary's Thistle
*   Green tea
*   Probiotics such as lactobacillus acidophilus and bifidobacterium
*   Selenium

Tenderstem (Brassica oleracea) is known as a "super vegetable". It is a cross between broccoli and Chinese kale. Tenderstem is high in immune boosting compounds such as glucosinolates, vitamins A, C and B6.

This is all available combined together in a powder called **"VKS Super Foods for Youngevity"**. This powder can be stirred into fresh juices or water to give you a quick energy and immune boosting effect. Typical serving sizes are 2 to 3 teaspoons twice daily. These super foods and herbs can help to revitalize sick and ageing cells, especially if the powder is stirred into fresh juices. After 4 weeks on this program you will see great benefits in your skin, energy levels and overall health.

For more information call the Health Advisory Service on (02) 4655 8855 and speak with one of Dr Sandra Cabot's naturopaths.

4. Increase the antioxidant content of your diet

Exposure to pollution, sunlight, stress, and just the processes of metabolism generate a lot of free radicals in our body. Free radical damage causes aging of our body, and can destroy cells and DNA; raising the risk of cancer. Therefore, it is wise to have as many antioxidants in our diet as possible.

ORAC stands for Oxygen Radical Absorbance Capacity, and it is a measure of the antioxidant capacity of foods. Dr. Guohua Cao, a physician and chemist at the Jean Mayer Human Nutrition Research Center on Aging at Tufts University, in Boston, developed the standardized ORAC assay. It measures the degree to which a food inhibits the action of an oxidizing agent and how long it takes to do so.

Top Antioxidant Foods

ORAC Units per 100 grams			
Vegetables		**Fruits**	
Kale	1,770	Prunes	5,770
Spinach	1,260	Raisins	2,830
Brussels sprouts	980	Blueberries	2,400
Broccoli	890	Blackberries	2,036
Beetroot	840	Strawberries	1,540
Red capsicum	710	Raspberries	1,220
Onion	450	Plums	949
Corn	400	Avocado	782
Eggplant	390	Oranges	750
Cauliflower	377	Red grapes	739
White potatoes	313	Cherries	670
Carrot	207	Kiwifruit	602

Prunes and raisins came out on top, but because they have been dehydrated, blueberries are actually the best antioxidant of all fruit and vegetables.

The Benefits of Juicing

Consuming fresh raw vegetable juices is one of the best ways to increase your antioxidant intake. Juices are a super concentrated supply of nutrients, phyto chemicals and enzymes. Ideally you would have juices on top of the vegetables and salads you already consume, not instead of. Because of their enzyme content and the fact that the vegetable matter has been crushed, juices are very easy on the digestive system; taking little effort to digest. Make sure you sip the juice very slowly, and dilute it if you find it too strong.

Selenium

This mineral is one of the most powerful antioxidants known. It is an essential component of the body's own antioxidant glutathione peroxidase. It acts to neutralize the by-products of metabolism, called free radicals. Several studies have indicated that selenium may help to protect the body against cancer. One such study found that men with prostate cancer had significantly lower blood selenium levels than men without prostate cancer. The study claims that low selenium is associated with a 4- to 5-fold increased risk of prostate cancer. Ref. 25.

Selenium is antagonistic to several toxic metals, including mercury, lead, arsenic, aluminium and cadmium. Selenium can bind with these metals and take them out of your body.

Selenium helps the body to fight viral infections such as hepatitis, Epstein Barr virus and cytomegalovirus. It has an anti-inflammatory action and helps to reduce the toxins generated in the body by viral infections and inflammation.

Carotenoids

These are a group of antioxidants found in brightly coloured fruits and vegetables. Studies have shown they act as antioxidants, and may help to protect us from cancer. Beta carotene is the most well known carotenoid; here are some others:

- **Lutein:** This is found in mangoes, corn, sweet potatoes, carrots, egg yolks and dark green leafy vegetables. Lutein is said to help protect us from developing cataracts and macular degeneration.

- **Zeaxanthin:** This is found in orange and yellow capsicum, oranges, corn, honeydew melon and egg yolks. Zeaxanthin is also involved in protecting the eyes from free radical damage, and conditions such as cataracts, glaucoma and macular degeneration.

- **Astaxanthin:** This carotenoid is found in orange and red fruit and vegetables, dark green leafy vegetables, as well as salmon, trout, prawns and red sea bream. It may protect us from the effects of the sun's ultraviolet light and enhance our immune system.

- **Lycopene:** This is found in red capsicum, watermelon, tomatoes, guava and pink grapefruit. Lycopene is best known for its protective effects against prostate cancer. Research has also shown it may protect us against lung, breast, gastrointestinal and endometrial cancers. Low blood lycopene levels may increase our risk of heart disease. Ref. 26.

4. Drink More Water

Many people do not drink enough water for optimal health. As a general rule we need between eight and ten glasses of pure water each day. Caffeine containing drinks and alcohol are diuretics, meaning they actually make your body lose water. Because tap water can be full of toxins, you are best off to drink purified, filtered, spring, mineral or distilled water. Initially, when you increase your water intake you may spend a lot of time dashing to the bathroom. This should lessen as your bladder becomes accustomed to holding more fluid. You can also minimize this inconvenience by drinking small sips of water throughout the day, rather than big gulps. We are often amazed when patients at our clinic tell us they do not have the time to drink water, when these people drink 6 cups of coffee each day. It takes much longer to make a cup of coffee and wait for it to cool down than it takes to drink a glass of water.

Here are some of the beneficial effects water has in our body:

- Maintains an optimal body temperature. In many cases, hot flushes can be reduced by increasing your water intake.

- Dilutes toxins and wastes, and facilitates their removal from the body. Remember that the liver converts fat soluble toxins into a water soluble form, ready for excretion in urine, perspiration, bile and the breath.

- Keeps our joints well lubricated.

- Softens the stool, preventing constipation.

- Improves energy and concentration

5. Move Your Body

Our bodies were designed to move. Sedentary lifestyles have
been blamed on conditions such as obesity, heart disease, diabetes,
arthritis and depression. It is important to make exercise a regular
part of your life, whether you are trying to lose weight or not.
Exercise is not a means to an end; it is important to exercise for the
rest of your life.

As toxins are being broken down and released, we want them to
make a quick exit; improving your circulation is one of the best
ways to do this. By pumping the blood around your body under
high pressure, your extremities will be cleansed with a fresh blood
supply. Perspiration is a great way of releasing toxins through
your skin. Exercise that makes you break out into a sweat is very
detoxifying; it is similar to the effects of a sauna.

 Just make sure you don't walk or jog along a busy street and
expose yourself to the pollution emanating from motor vehicles.
**Here are some other reasons to get off your butt and get
moving:**

- Exercise speeds up your metabolic rate; helping you
  to lose weight more easily.

- It lowers your resting heart rate; therefore your heart
  will not have to work as hard to pump blood around
  your body.

- It improves your circulation.

- Exercise helps to normalize your blood pressure.

- It improves your cholesterol levels; helping to lower LDL (bad) cholesterol and increase HDL (good) cholesterol.

- Exercise enhances the function of the immune system.

- It improves insulin sensitivity; reducing your chances of developing
Syndrome X and diabetes.

- Exercise increases muscular strength, stamina and endurance.

- It improves your balance and flexibility, reducing the risk of falls.

- By strengthening the muscles surrounding your joints, you will be protecting your joints from damage.

- Exercise lessens anxiety and depression. Numerous studies have shown exercise is just as beneficial for mild to moderate depression as antidepressant medication.

- Exercise helps you to cope better with stress.

- It can improve the quality of your sleep.

- Exercise reduces cravings and improves the resolve to lose weight when dieting.

- Exercise makes you feel good about yourself.

- Exercise is triumph over laziness.

6. Include Natural Antibiotics In Your Diet

Many easily obtained foods and herbs have powerful immune boosting and infection fighting properties. Try to include as many of these in your diet as possible regularly. Some of the best antibiotics are listed below:

• **Garlic** is one of the most powerful antibiotics. Once garlic is chopped or crushed, the active component allicin is formed. Allicin has antibacterial, antifungal and antiparasitic activity. Studies have shown garlic to be effective against Candida, Giardia, Entamoeba histolytica, H. pylori and Staphylococcus aureus. Ref. 27. Populations that consume a lot of garlic have lower rates of cancer and cardiovascular disease. Cooking garlic damages some of the therapeutic principles, so it is best eaten raw.

• **Onion** and **Cruciferous vegetables** (broccoli, cabbage) contain organosulfur. These natural sulfur compounds have antibiotic and antifungal properties. Another form of organic sulfur you can include in your diet is called Methyl Sulfonyl Methane (MSM). This compound assists your immune system to fight infections and is needed for phase 2 detoxification by the liver. MSM can be obtained as a supplement in powder form.

• **Olive Leaf.** The active ingredient in olive leaf is oleuropein. Studies have shown that olive leaf has antibacterial, antifungal and antiviral properties. Ref. 28. Olive leaf is excellent for the symptoms of colds and flu, as well as gastrointestinal, respiratory and urinary tract infections. Olive leaf extract can be taken in capsule form or as a liquid. It is more effective when combined with another powerful immune boosting herb call Andrographis paniculata, and zinc.

• **Coconut oil** is rich in lauric acid, which studies have demonstrated is antiviral, antibacterial and antifungal; it is excellent for the immune system. Coconut fat has received a lot of bad publicity because it is high in saturated fat, but we now know that the fats in coconut are medium chain triglycerides; these do not raise cholesterol or contribute to heart disease. Clinical trials are currently being done on the effectiveness of lauric acid in lowering the viral load in HIV/AIDS patients. Include coconut milk and coconut cream in your cooking. If you use coconut fat for cooking or as a dressing, make sure you purchase unrefined oil such as the Melrose Organic Coconut Oil brand.

The anti-parasitic herbs Berberis, wormwood and thyme have many antibiotic properties also. You can read more about them on page 77.

7. Increase The Fibre In Your Diet

Fibre is the part of complex carbohydrates that cannot be digested by us. Therefore, it passes right through our body. Fibre does not provide nutrients in our diet; it has other benefits such as:

- Increased bowel transit time; therefore reducing the tendency to constipation, and the risk of colon cancer.

- It helps to lower cholesterol and triglyceride levels by binding with them in the gut; inhibiting their re-absorption.

- Fibre slows the absorption of sugar into the bloodstream, thereby lowering the glycemic index of the food you have eaten.

- Fibre slows the absorption of fat you have eaten, helping to keep you full for longer.

- Certain types of fibre swell in the digestive tract, increasing the satiety of a meal.

Fibre can be classified as soluble or insoluble.
Insoluble fibre increases the weight, bulk and softness of the stool. Good sources of insoluble fibre are whole grains, fruit and

vegetables.

Soluble fibre dissolves in water to form a thick, gummy solution. It is particularly good for lowering cholesterol, slowing the absorption of sugar into the bloodstream and binding with toxins in our gut. Good sources of soluble fibre are seaweed, oats, rice, legumes, pectin in fruit and vegetables and legumes. Slippery elm, psyllium and LSA are rich in soluble fibre.

When increasing the quantity of fibre in your diet, make sure you start slowly. Too much fibre added too quickly can lead to bloating, gas and cramps. Whenever you increase your fibre intake, you must increase your water intake, otherwise the fibre will dry up in your gut and worsen constipation.

We will now look at the specific benefits of some types of soluble fibre:

- **PECTIN**

Rich sources of pectin include apples, bananas, grapes, cherries, pineapple, avocados, raisins and carob.

Pectin is particularly good at helping to lower blood cholesterol levels. The liver pumps excess cholesterol into the bile, which then enters the intestines. If pectin is present in your intestines, it will bind with the cholesterol and take it out of your body.

Pectin changes into galacturonic acid, which can combine with heavy metals such as lead and mercury in the gut, and take them out of your body. Pectin can also combine with the radio active substance strontium 90, and take it out of the body.

- **SEAWEED**

There are many different kinds of sea vegetables, yet most people would not be aware of them. You may have eaten sushi that is wrapped in nori, and ice cream you have eaten probably contained seaweed extract as an emulsifier. Sea vegetables are an extremely rich source of minerals such as calcium, potassium, iron, magnesium and iodine. All of these minerals support healthy thyroid function and strong bones. Seaweed is also rich in antioxidants, phyto nutrients and antiviral properties.

Seaweeds are great detoxifiers. The brown seaweeds such as

kombu and arame contain alginic acid. This is able to bind to heavy metals, radioactive substances and other toxins in the gut, carrying them out of the body via bowel motions. Studies have shown that eating seaweed regularly can cleanse our body of over 50% of these toxins.

Common varieties of seaweed include nori, kombu, arame, agar-agar, dulse, and kelp. You should be able to find at least some of these sea vegetables in dehydrated form in health food stores, and even the health section of good supermarkets. Most types of seaweed need to be soaked in water for a period of time before use. You can then add them to soups, stews, casseroles and salads.

8. Support Your Lymphatic System

Since the lymphatic fluid is not pumped around the body like the blood is pumped around by the heart, muscular contractions are required to move lymph. Exercise has an incredibly cleansing effect on the lymphatic system by improving its circulation.

Dairy products can congest your lymphatic system. If you suffer with fluid retention, sinusitis, post nasal drip, hayfever, asthma or excessive mucus, you may benefit from removing dairy products from your diet; these include cow's milk and all products containing it. The protein in dairy products is called casein, and in sensitive individuals it can stimulate the production of histamine and mucus. Better alternatives to cow's milk are rice, soy, oat, almond, coconut, goat or sheep milk. Excessive fats in your diet, especially partially hydrogenated vegetable oil can clog the tiny lymph vessels in the intestines called the lacteals.

Saunas and steam baths are very powerful ways to drive toxins out of your body. Research has even shown that saunas can remove pesticides and heavy metals from the body. Ref. 29. Some people notice a chemical smell on their body when they have a sauna. Unlike Finland, where just about every home has a sauna; in this country you will probably have to rely on gyms and health spas. Make sure you drink plenty of water before and after having a sauna or steam bath, because you will lose a lot of water in the process.

Dry skin brushing is another way to stimulate lymphatic flow. Before you enter the shower or bath, use a loofah or body mitt to vigorously slough the dead skin cells from your body. Make your brushing movements towards the major lymph nodes in the body; in the arm pits and groin areas. Lymphatic drainage massage works on this principle, but at a deeper level.

9. Avoid a High Intake Of Sugar and Refined Carbohydrate

An excessive sugar intake long term will weaken your immune system and make you much more prone to infections. Sugar feeds harmful bacteria, yeast and fungi in the body. Excess sugar in your digestive tract can promote bloating, gas, cramps and Candida overgrowth. Long term high sugar intake can promote weight gain and make you more susceptible to diabetes.

Sugar can leave you mineral deficient. The minerals needed to digest sugar are chromium, manganese, cobalt, copper, zinc, and magnesium. These minerals have been stripped from the sugar cane in the refining process. This forces your body to deplete its own mineral reserves to process the sugar. Raw sugar, brown sugar and honey are very slightly higher in mineral content, yet they still act as sugar in your body.

People with Syndrome X often have strong cravings for sugar and refined carbohydrates and are overweight. If this is you, the book "Can't Lose Weight? You Could Have Syndrome X" will give you valuable information.

If you like the taste of sweet foods and beverages, use the natural, herbal sweetener stevia instead. This comes in liquid, powder and tablet form. You can use it to sweeten coffee, tea and even use it in your cooking. Stevia is an herb that grows traditionally in South America and has been used there for hundreds of years. It has been used commercially in Japan for the last 30 years. Stevia has no effect on blood sugar or insulin levels, and is calorie free. **For more information about stevia please call our Health Advisory Service on 02 4655 8855.**

Chapter Seven

DIETARY GUIDELINES FOR THE 2 WEEK DETOX

Dietary Guidelines For The 2-Week Detox

You must follow these dietary principles in order to achieve a deep cleansing:

Avoid the following:

- Dairy products, this means no cow, goat or sheep milk, or any products containing these.

- Gluten. This is found in wheat, rye, oats, spelt, kamut, triticale and barley, and all foods containing these. Gluten is hidden in many foods, so you will need to read food labels carefully.

- Red meat, fish, chicken and eggs. You will be obtaining protein from vegetarian sources such as grains, legumes, nuts and seeds.

- Sugar and foods that contain added sugar.

- Alcohol.

- Coffee.

- Food additives such as artificial colours, flavours, preservatives, artificial sweeteners, MSG, etc.

- Vegetable oil that does not state cold pressed, or extra virgin; margarine; partially hydrogenated or hydrogenated vegetable oil.

You should include the following:

- Two litres of pure water each day. This may include spring water, mineral water, filtered water or distilled water.
- One or two glasses of raw vegetable juice each day.
- You may include regular tea, green tea and herbal teas in your diet.
  Tea should be free of sugar, artificial sweeteners and dairy milk. You can use stevia to sweeten your tea.

- You may include sea salt in your cooking; it is preferable to regular table salt.
- Beneficial fats, such as those found in olive oil, flaxseed oil, avocados, coconut milk and raw, unsalted nuts and seeds.
- The "Detox Soup" should form one meal each day during the two week detox. You may have it for breakfast, lunch or dinner.
- You must have one raw vegetable salad each day, either for lunch or dinner. You can make up your own simple salad, or use one of our recipes.
- Take a good antioxidant supplement and liver tonic. While you are detoxing, your liver and fatty tissues will be releasing stored toxins in large quantities. Hence, it is important to take the right supplements in order to protect your tissues from damage they may incur in the process. The right supplements can also help to protect you from experiencing some unpleasant symptoms of rapid detoxification, such as nausea, headaches and aches and pains.

An antioxidant containing selenium, vitamin E, zinc and vitamin C should be taken daily. These vitamins and minerals can be obtained combined in the one tablet.

A good liver tonic should contain St Mary's Thistle, green tea extract and various amino acids and vitamins. You can read more about liver tonics on page 85. If you are prone to constipation or sluggish bowels, you may need a bulk laxative made of rice and soy bran and pectin, to mop up the toxins that enter your intestines.

For more information about antioxidants, liver tonics and fibre supplements, please call our Health Advisory on 02 4655 8855.

Cooking Tips

In the following recipes, you may encounter foods you have never eaten before. All of them can be found in the health isle of a good supermarket, or in a health food store. There are no ingredients you must use for this detox program to be effective. If a particular ingredient is unavailable in your area, out of season, too expensive, or you do not like its taste, it is fine to avoid it, or substitute with another food you do enjoy. Many of these recipes contain spices; if you don't like them you can avoid them. The recipes in this book are merely suggestions. If you are short of time, or following recipes is not your thing, it is fine to come up with your own combinations, as long as you follow the guidelines above. You could make a simple salad; throw in some tinned legumes, such as four bean mix, and a handful of raw nuts and seeds. You could dress this with olive oil and lemon juice and it could be a simple, quick lunch. If you would like to be more creative with your meals, we have some recipes for you on the following pages.

Here are some tips to help you out when shopping and preparing meals:

• **Tamari.** This is a wheat free soy sauce; you should find it alongside the regular soy sauce in the health section of supermarkets.
• **Non-dairy milk.** You may use soy, rice, almond or coconut milk. Make sure the milk is gluten free; malt extract and maltodextrin are common sources of gluten. Milk that is malt free, or sweetened with rice malt is fine.

• **Legumes.** The easiest way to cook with legumes is to use the tinned ones that are already cooked. Try to find a brand that does not contain artificial additives. Suitable brands include Bio Nature, Eden, Annalisa, Goya, Gustini, Rosa, Valverde, QuickPulse and McKenzies.
You may purchase dried legumes, however they will need to be soaked overnight, rinsed and then cooked for approximately 30

minutes in fresh water.

• **Gluten free grains.** You are able to eat brown rice, corn, quinoa, amaranth and millet. These grains are increasingly available in supermarkets and health food stores. You can buy rice flakes and cook them like porridge. A suitable brand is Lowans Rice Flakes. Follow the cooking instructions on the packet.

Quinoa was one of the staple foods of the Incas, and grows traditionally in the South American Andes. Quinoa has the highest protein content of any grain. It is also a rich source of calcium, iron, B vitamins, phosphorus, and vitamin E. You can find whole quinoa or quinoa flakes in stores.

Amaranth is an ancient grain consumed by the Aztecs. Amaranth is also high in protein, particularly the amino acid lysine, which is deficient in most grains. Amaranth is also high in calcium, magnesium, silicon and vitamin C. You may find puffed amaranth in stores that you can use as a breakfast cereal.

Spelt, kamut and triticale cannot be consumed because they contain gluten. You may eat gluten free bread, pasta, cereals and muesli.

• **Seaweed.** Many varieties of seaweed are now available in health food stores, the health section, or Asian food section of supermarkets. Seaweed has powerful detoxification properties, and is high in minerals. Eating seaweed is not a compulsory part of this detox; if you cannot obtain it, seaweed may be omitted from the recipes.

• **Nut butters/pastes.** If you eat peanut butter, choose a brand that is 100% peanuts, with no other ingredients, such as the Sanitarium brand. You may also eat almond, hazelnut, cashew or macadamia butter. Tahini is the paste made from ground sesame seeds; it is a major component of hummus.

• **LSA.** This is a combination of ground linseeds, sunflower seeds and almonds. It is a tasty source of protein and Essential Fatty Acids that can be added to smoothies or dips, or sprinkled over fresh fruit or cereals. LSA can be purchased from stores, or you can make it yourself. The recipe is below:

3 cups linseeds (flaxseeds)
2 cups sunflower seeds
1 cup almonds

For smaller quantities you can use tablespoons instead of cups. Grind the ingredients together in a coffee grinder or food processor to a fine meal. Store in an airtight container in the fridge or freezer.

• **Sea salt.** This is preferable to ordinary table salt because it contains a range of minerals, and does not contain aluminium as an anti-caking agent.

Cautions To Consider Before Detoxing

Do not discontinue any medications that were prescribed to you by your doctor.
If you are a diabetic and take medication, you should monitor your blood sugar regularly while on this program, and be supervised by your own doctor. Your requirement for medication may change.
Do not follow this detox if you suffer with kidney failure or liver failure.
Do not follow this detox if you are pregnant or breastfeeding. Removing toxins from your body can leave them ending up in your baby's circulation. Hence, do not follow this program if you are pregnant or breast feeding.
Consult with your doctor before following this detox if you are undergoing treatment for cancer.

To Fast Or Not To Fast

Abstaining from all food is not recommended for a number of reasons. Fasting causes an extremely rapid release of toxins from the tissues into the bloodstream. This can make you feel quite unwell. When your liver is working hard to process toxins it needs a good supply of nutrients and antioxidants to mop up the free radicals generated in the process. If you don't eat anything, and don't take antioxidant supplements, the free radicals can cause a great deal of tissue damage.

Due to high sugar and carbohydrate diets, blood sugar imbalances are common. Conditions such as hypoglycaemia and diabetes are contraindications for fasting.

Symptoms Of Rapid Detoxification

If detoxification is carried out too rapidly, or if you have accumulated a lot of toxins, you may experience some unpleasant symptoms when they are released. These could include the following:

• **Headaches** are very common, and usually occur if you have given up or reduced your caffeine intake. Caffeine causes constriction of the blood vessels in your brain; in the absence of caffeine the blood vessels can dilate, triggering a headache. Headaches may be unrelated to caffeine intake, and just part of the detoxification also.
Make sure you are drinking at least 2 litres of water each day. Try some pure lavender oil on your temples and a neck massage before resorting to painkillers.

• **Increased urination.** This may occur as a result of your increased water intake, and be an early symptom of weight loss. It is a good sign because you will be removing a great deal of water soluble toxins through your kidneys, and getting rid of fluid retention. This diet removes common food allergens, thus will help with fluid retention also.

• **Cravings.** In the early stages of this detox plan you will probably find yourself craving sugar and refined carbohydrates. This is natural because sugar is addictive, and you will miss it at first. If you suffer with a Candida yeast infection you will find yourself craving sugar. Also, foods you may be allergic to such as wheat and dairy products can be addictive, and you will not be consuming these. The cravings will definitely pass within a few days. Make sure you are drinking enough water, eating enough protein, such as nuts, seeds and legumes, and consuming good fats in your diet such as olive oil and avocados.

• **Change in bowel habits.** This is common with a change of diet. Because you will probably be including more fibre in your diet, you may experience temporary bloating and flatulence. This should pass soon; make sure you eat slowly, chew well and don't drink too much water at meal times. Sipping on a little water with apple cider vinegar before meals should help your digestion. You may also notice more frequent bowel movements; this is good because more toxins will be excreted through your liver and bowels. Again this should settle down soon.

• **Skin eruptions.** If you suffer with acne, you may experience a temporary aggravation of the condition, as the skin is given a greater toxin load to excrete.

• **Generalized aches and pains,** and flu like symptoms may occur in some people. This just means your body needs to rest more, so please take it easy and try to get more sleep.

Chapter Eight

RECIPES TO DETOX YOUR BODY

Breakfast Meal Ideas

• Gluten free muesli with soy, rice, almond or diluted coconut milk. You can add chopped fresh fruit or grated apple to the muesli. Make sure the milk is gluten free. Suitable brands of muesli include Healtheries, Freedom Foods, Monster Muesli or Mellow Yellow.

- Rice porridge with soy, almond, rice or diluted coconut milk. You can use Lowans Rice Flakes. Ground LSA can be sprinkled on the porridge for added fibre.

If you can find puffed amaranth, whole or flaked quinoa in a supermarket or health food store, these grains can also be used to make porridge.

- Two pieces of toast made from gluten free bread. Suitable toppings include:
  - **avocado**
  - **hummus**
  - **tahini**
  - **almond, cashew, hazelnut or macadamia butter**
  - **baked beans (ensure these are gluten free)**
  - **nut butter with banana**

Suitable brands of gluten free bread include R & R Bakery Products, Lifestyle Bakery, Pav's Allergy Bakery.

If you prefer, you can use rice cakes or Corn Thins instead of the bread.

Sample 2 Week Menu

Upon rising, drink a glass of pure water with the juice of half a lemon or lime. In winter you may use warm water with a teaspoon of freshly grated ginger.

You may drink a glass of raw vegetable juice before breakfast, or if it is more convenient, have it in the evening when you come home from work.

What About Serving Sizes?

In many of the recipes serving sizes have not been included. This detox is not specifically a weight loss diet, therefore, you are to eat according to your appetite. You should not be feeling hungry or weak on this program. If your job or lifestyle are physically demanding, or you are male, it is fine to eat more.

WEEK ONE

Monday

Breakfast
- 1 bowl gluten free muesli with 1 chopped pear and non-dairy milk.

Lunch
- 1 bowl detox soup with salad of your choice or fresh fruit of your choice.

Dinner
- Cauliflower pasta, see recipe pg. 141 with a garden salad.

Tuesday

Breakfast
- 1 bowl rice porridge with 1 tablespoon of LSA sprinkled on top, with non-dairy milk. Add fruit of your choice.

Lunch
- Mixed bean salad, see recipe pg. 164 served with brown rice.

Dinner
- 1 bowl detox soup with salad or fruit.

Wednesday

Breakfast
- 2 pieces gluten free toast with baked beans and one

piece of fruit.

Lunch
- Herbed lentils see recipe pg. 146 served with brown rice and a small salad.

Dinner
- 1 bowl detox soup with salad or fruit.

Thursday

Breakfast
- 2 pieces gluten free toast, one spread with avocado, the other with almond butter. One piece of fruit.

Lunch
- 1 bowl detox soup with salad or fruit.

Dinner
- Detox Shepherd's Pie; see recipe pg. 153, served with Avocado and Sunflower salad, see recipe pg. 163.

Friday

Breakfast
- Breakfast Polenta, see recipe pg. 125.

Lunch
- Spicy vegetables in coconut milk, see recipe pg. 143, served with brown rice and a salad.

Dinner
- 1 bowl detox soup with salad or fruit.

Saturday

Breakfast
- 2 pieces gluten free toast spread with hummus. One piece of fruit.

Lunch
- 1 bowl detox soup with salad or fruit.

Dinner
- Quinoa Pilaf, see recipe pg. 147, served with Garden salad with avocado dressing, see recipe pg. 159.

Sunday

Breakfast
- A bowl of fresh fruit salad sprinkled with 2 tablespoons of LSA.

Lunch
- 1 bowl detox soup with salad or fruit.

Dinner
- Cannellini bean patties, see recipe pg. 138, served with a salad.

WEEK TWO

Monday

Breakfast
- 1 glass Classic Banana smoothie, see recipe pg. 127.

Lunch
- Mediterranean pasta with olives , see recipe pg. 142, served

with Rena's Red Kohlrabi salad, see recipe pg. 158.

Dinner
- 1 bowl detox soup with salad or fruit.

Tuesday

Breakfast
- 2 pieces gluten free bread or rice, or corn crackers topped with banana and tahini. One piece of fruit.

Lunch
- 1 bowl detox soup with salad or fruit.

Dinner
- Baked Nutty Vegetables, see recipe pg. 139, served with a salad.

Wednesday

Breakfast
- 1 bowl gluten free muesli with non-dairy milk and fresh fruit.

Lunch
- Rice with red lentils, see recipe pg. 148, served with Avocado salad, see recipe pg. 161.

Dinner
- 1 bowl detox soup with salad or fruit.

Thursday

Breakfast
- 1 bowl rice porridge with non-dairy milk, topped with sliced strawberries or other berries.

Detox your body and save your health

Lunch
- Sandwich using gluten free bread, with hummus, grated carrot and sultanas.

Dinner
- 1 bowl detox soup, served with a salad or fresh fruit.

Friday

Breakfast
- 1 glass Passionate Passionfruit smoothie, see recipe pg. 126.

Lunch
- 1 bowl detox soup with a salad or fresh fruit.

Dinner
- Spicy Bean Risotto, see recipe pg. 136, served with Carrot salad, see recipe pg. 160.

Saturday

Breakfast
- 1 bowl quinoa or rice porridge with non-dairy milk. Top with grated apple, cinnamon and chopped walnuts.

Lunch
- 1 bowl detox soup served with salad or fresh fruit.

Dinner
- Chick pea curry, see recipe pg. 137, served with gluten free pasta and a salad.

Sunday

Breakfast
- Scrambled tofu, see recipe pg. 125. Serve with fresh fruit.

Lunch
- 1 bowl detox soup served with salad or fresh fruit.

Dinner
- Black Eyed Beans with Spinach, see recipe pg. 150, served with Rice and Sesame Salad, see recipe pg. 163.

Snacks

If you are hungry, you may have two snacks each day, such as at morning tea and afternoon tea, or after dinner. Here are some ideas for healthy detox snacks:

- Fresh fruit.
- Raw, un-roasted, unsalted nuts and seeds, such as Brazil nuts, hazelnuts, almonds, pecans, walnuts, cashews, pine nuts, macadamias, pepitas, sunflower seeds, sesame seeds.
- Vegetable sticks served with hummus, tahini, nut butter or salsa.
- Gluten free crackers/cakes topped with:

    - Avocado, sliced tomato & parsley
    - Hummus with grated carrot
    - Tahini with chopped dates
    - Nut butter with banana
    - Banana sprinkled with sesame seeds

Raw Juice Recipes

The consumption of raw vegetable juices is an essential part of our detox program. Please consume one to two glasses of raw juice each day. Store bought bottled or tinned juice is not suitable, because it is not a raw juice. It is best to consume the juice as soon as it is made, as exposure to air will start to destroy the enzymes and nutrients found in the vegetables. Also, you must sip the juice slowly in order to digest it properly. Gulping vegetable juices can lead to flatulence and loose stools.

When making juices, it is preferable to use predominantly vegetables, rather than fruit. Vegetables are usually higher in mineral content, and they are lower in sugars, or carbohydrate. If you are interested in weight loss, it is best to limit the amount of fruit, carrot and beetroot in your juices.

Of the following recipes, you can choose which juice is most applicable for you, or you can alternate between all of these juices.

Bowel Cleansing Juice

1 handful chicory leaves
1 green apple with skin
2 fresh or dried figs (if dried soak in water overnight)
1 pear with skin
½ beetroot
1 clove garlic

Apples are high in pectin, which is a great source of soluble fibre. Figs and pears are a great source of fibre. Beetroot is a powerful detoxifier and can help with constipation.
Garlic is anti-microbial and anti-parasitic. Chicory is a bitter vegetable, stimulating the liver to produce bile; which acts as a natural laxative.

Liver Detoxifier

1 handful chicory leaves
2 cabbage leaves
1 carrot
¼ red onion
1 cup broccoli flowerets
2 red radishes

Chicory stimulates the liver to produce bile. Cabbage, broccoli and onion are high in natural sulphur compounds; needed by the liver for phase two detoxification. Onion also contains natural infection fighting properties.
Carrot is high in antioxidants, needed to mop up free radicals produced as a result of liver detoxification. Radishes are excellent liver and gallbladder cleansers, helping to reduce the risk of gallstone formation.

Kidney Cleanser

2 sticks celery
4 sticks asparagus
Thick slice watermelon
Handful green beans
1 clove garlic

Celery and watermelon are natural diuretics; celery also helps the kidneys to excrete excess acids. Asparagus reduces the risk of kidney stones by helping to break up oxalic acid crystals in the kidneys. Green beans are used to strengthen the kidneys and liver in Oriental medicine.
Garlic is a natural antibiotic, helping to fight infections.

Infection Fighter

½ red onion
1 clove garlic
½ cm fresh ginger
3 red radishes
1 carrot
½ cup blueberries
2 cabbage leaves

Garlic contains allicin, which helps to fight infections. Onion and ginger contain infection fighting properties.
Radish acts as a natural antibiotic, and helps to clear mucus from the body. Radish and cabbage contain natural sulphur compounds, which help to fight infections.
Carrots and blueberries are high in antioxidants, which have immune enhancing properties.

Lymphatic Cleanser

2 sticks celery
1 carrot
½ red onion
1 handful parsley
1 slice pineapple
3 red radishes

Celery and parsley are natural diuretics, helping with fluid retention. Pineapple has anti inflammatory properties and reduces mucus congestion. Onion and radish are high in natural sulphur compounds and help to boost circulation.
Carrot helps to reduce inflammation and mucus in the body.

Weight Loss Juice

1 slice pineapple
1 grapefruit, peeled
½ cm fresh ginger
1 handful chicory leaves
2 cabbage leaves
2 Brussels sprouts

Brussels sprouts help insulin to work better in the body, improving Syndrome X. Pineapple acts as a mild diuretic and laxative. Grapefruit assists liver function and fat burning. Chicory and cabbage assist the liver with fat burning. Ginger helps to improve circulation.
If you take medication, check with your doctor whether grapefruit interacts with it.

Skin Clearer

2 apricots
1 carrot
1 green apple
1 handful endive
1 slice lemon
1 handful parsley
Apricots and carrots are high in minerals and beta carotene, helping to strengthen connective tissue. Apple improves the elimination of toxins via the gut, reducing their elimination via the skin.
Endive and parsley are liver tonics, promoting the secretion of bile, which has a cleansing effect. Lemon has natural antibiotic properties, helping to prevent infections.

Lung Tonic Juice

1 slice pineapple
½ red onion
1 clove garlic
1 red apple
3 red radishes

Pineapple is great for reducing mucus congestion, helping with conditions such as asthma, bronchitis, sinusitis and post nasal drip. Onion and garlic contain antibiotic properties, which act in the lungs as they are excreted in the breath.
Apples are high in silicon, which helps to strengthen the connective tissue of the lungs. Radishes help to clear mucus from the respiratory tract.

Breakfast Recipes

You may choose a breakfast from one of the Breakfast Choices on page 112, or use one of the recipes below:

- ## Breakfast Polenta

Serves 2

Ingredients

1 cup polenta
4 cups water
½ cup prunes, chopped, or other dried fruit
¼ tsp stevia powder or 1 drop liquid stevia
¼ tsp cinnamon powder
1 tsp grated fresh ginger (optional)
½ cup chopped pecans

Method

Cook the polenta in the water according to packet directions. Once cooked, stir in the remaining ingredients and serve.

- ## Scrambled Tofu

Serves 4

Ingredients

1 onion, finely diced
1 red capsicum, finely chopped
2 tsp olive oil
1 tsp turmeric
½ tsp cumin

2 packets firm tofu, crumbled
Tamari to taste

Method

Sauté the onion and spices in olive oil for 3-5 minutes. Add the capsicum and cook a further 3 minutes. Add the crumbled tofu and cook covered for 10-15 minutes. It may need occasional stirring.

- **Fresh Fruit Salad sprinkled with 2 tablespoons of LSA.**

- **Passionate Passionfruit Smoothie.**

Ingredients

1 cup soy, almond or rice milk
Pulp from 1 passionfruit
2 Tbsp LSA

Blend together and serve immediately.

- ### Berry Smoothie

Ingredients

1 cup soy, almond or rice milk
½ cup blueberries
2 Tbsp hazelnut butter/paste

Blend together well and serve immediately.

- ### Classic Banana Smoothie

Ingredients

1 cup soy, almond or rice milk
1 frozen banana
¼ tsp stevia powder or 1 drop liquid stevia
2 Tbsp LSA

Blend together and serve immediately.

Main Course Recipes

DETOX SOUP
(Adapted from a family recipe of the well-known Italian Minestrone).

This soup must be consumed as one of your meals each day for the duration of the detox. You may have it for breakfast, lunch or dinner. You could make a large amount on the weekends, or when you have more time, and consume leftovers during the week.

The soup is cooked in 40 –45 minutes. The ingredients must be added in the specific order as mentioned below.
The ingredients could be varied at will to include seasonal vegetables. The essential ingredients are highlighted in bold. If you really dislike an ingredient, leave it out.
The water content could be increased if preferred. The following recipe uses 5 litres of water in a 5-litre saucepan.

INGREDIENTS: (in order of preparation and as they are added in a 5-litre saucepan)
Note: The time between stages is the time taken to prepare, chop and add the various ingredients. The soup freezes well.

Stage 1-(15 minutes): STOVE on MEDIUM HEAT:
2 Tbsp **cold pressed olive oil**, a large **onion** finely chopped,
Stir frequently till onion is glassy.
ADD: 30 mm grated fresh **ginger**, fresh continental **parsley** finely chopped, 1 tsp **turmeric**, 2 small **tomatoes** cubed, ½ turnip and ½ parsnip finely chopped, one grated **carrot**, 1 cup cubed **pumpkin**, 1 cubed zucchini, a large cubed **potato**.
Stir.
Stage 2-(Approximately 15 minutes): Increase temperature to MEDIUM HIGH.

ADD: 2 cups of water and 2 Tbsp tamari, 2 Brussels sprouts finely chopped, 2 cups of chopped cauliflower, a chopped broccoli floweret, a chopped **silver beet**: stalk and leaf, 420gr tin garden **peas** or 500gr frozen **peas**. If you like, you can add garlic, green beans, pre-soaked green lentils and bok choy.
Stir.

Stage 3-(Approximately 10 or more minutes)
ADD: 184gr tin of champignon pieces and stems, 1 cup English spinach, fresh or frozen, five strips Alaria, (wild Atlantic wakame), 5 strips **Dulse** (wild Atlantic Sea vegetable) and 3 Tbsp Genmai or Mugi **Miso** (seasoning). The seaweed should be soaked in water for 15 minutes and rinsed before being added to the soup.
1 tsp ground **nutmeg**.
ADD: 4 cups of water and return to boil.
Stir.
Reduce to SIMMER until the vegetables are cooked.
Keep the lid on and turn the stove off.

More pumpkin, tomatoes and/or potato can be added to make a thicker soup.

Benefits Of The Detox Soup

The essential ingredients of the detox soup have been chosen specifically for their therapeutic properties.

• **Cold pressed olive oil**, also known, as extra virgin olive oil is high in monounsaturated fat; this makes it more stable when heated to high temperatures. Extra virgin olive oil is not extracted using heat, and it has not been refined, therefore the beneficial fatty acids have not been destroyed, and the antioxidants remain in the oil.

• **Onion** is a rich source of antioxidants, sulfur compounds, vitamin C, potassium, and folate (folic acid). One antioxidant found in onions is quercetin; this substance has an anti inflammatory and anti allergic effect in the body. Onions have a blood thinning effect, helping to reduce the risk of blood clots.

• **Ginger** has been used in Asian food and medicine for thousands of years. It has anti inflammatory properties, helping with arthritis and menstrual cramps. Ginger acts as a natural antibiotic in the body, and helps to settle the digestion; helping with indigestion and motion sickness.

• **Parsley** is a member of the carrot family, and is an extremely good source of iron. It is an excellent diuretic and can help to reduce the tendency to form kidney stones.

• **Turmeric** is a bright yellow spice and a major component of curry powder. It is related to ginger, but much milder tasting. A lot of research has been done on the benefits of the active component of turmeric, called curcumin. Studies have shown that turmeric has antioxidant, anti inflammatory and anti cancer effects. It promotes better stage two detoxification in the liver cells. Chinese researchers have shown that curcumin exerts suppressive effects on human breast cancer cells through a number of mechanisms. Ref. 30.

Recent studies have also shown that curcumin can help protect against the development of Alzheimer's disease. It does this by reducing the buildup of amyloid protein plaques; common in the brains of those with Alzheimer's disease. Ref. 31.
Include turmeric in your diet as often as possible.

• **Tomatoes** are a rich source of vitamin C, beta carotene and potassium. The red pigment in tomatoes is the antioxidant lycopene. Numerous studies have shown that it can help to protect against prostate cancer, as well as rectal, colon, lung and breast cancer. The lycopene is absorbed better if the tomatoes are eaten with some fat, such as the olive oil in this recipe.

• **Carrot and Pumpkin** are both excellent sources of beta carotene, which is converted into vitamin A in the body. Vitamin A is needed for healthy skin, hair and eyes. Pumpkin is also a good source of silicon. Carrots are a great source of chlorine and sulphur, both needed by the liver for detoxification.

• **Potato** is a great source of potassium, magnesium, sulphur and silicon. Potatoes are soothing to the stomach and intestines.

• **Silverbeet** is a rich source of carotenoids and folic acid.

• **Peas** belong to the legume family and are a rich source of protein. They are also high in fibre, helping to eliminate toxins via the gut; as well as phosphorus and iron.

• **Dulse** is a blue and red pigmented seaweed that grows in flat, smooth fronds shaped like mittens. It is extremely concentrated in iodine, and is also very rich in manganese. Like all seaweeds, dulse is able to absorb toxins such as heavy metals and radioactive substances in the gut and take them out of the body. It also helps to lower cholesterol levels via a similar action.

• **Miso** is a fermented soybean paste thought to have originated in China approximately 2,500 years ago. It is made by combining cooked soybeans, a healthy mould (koji), grains such as brown rice or barley, and sea salt. Miso ranges in colour from a dark brown to a creamy beige. This recipe calls for a light coloured, mild tasting miso.

All miso is a good source of protein and contains some beneficial bacteria like in yoghurt. According to Oriental traditions, miso promotes good health and a long life, can help to treat radiation sickness, and neutralizes some of the harmful effects of cigarette smoke and air pollution. Ref. 32.

• **Nutmeg** is a spice with a variety of healing properties; it can help insomnia, anxiety, indigestion, diarrhoea and joint pain. Nutmeg may also help to lower blood pressure, lower cholesterol, and improve circulation. Ingesting too much nutmeg (between one and three whole nuts) can produce nausea, hallucinations, swelling and shock.

The following recipes can be used for either lunch or dinner.

Rice Noodles with Chili Vegetables

You should find rice noodles in the Asian food section of your supermarket.

Serves 4

Ingredients

1 Tbsp olive oil
1 onion, chopped
2 garlic cloves, finely chopped (optional)
1 red chili, seeded & finely chopped (optional)
1 red capsicum, finely diced
4 medium button squash, chopped

8 baby sweetcorn, chopped
400g can borlotti beans, rinsed & drained
1 can diced tinned tomatoes
1 Tbsp tamari
2 Tbsp chopped fresh coriander
Sea salt & black pepper to taste

Method

Cook the garlic, onion and chili in olive oil for 5 minutes. Stir
in the other vegetables, beans, tamari, salt and pepper. Bring to
the boil, then simmer covered for 30 minutes. If it is too watery,
leave the lid off to allow excess water to evaporate. Cook the rice
noodles according to packet directions. Spoon the noodles onto
serving plates, top with the vegetable mixture, and garnish with
fresh coriander.

Rice Pilaf

Serves 4

Ingredients

Wild rice is available alongside regular rice in most supermarkets.

225g mixed brown and wild rice
15 mL olive oil
1 onion, chopped
2 cloves garlic, finely chopped (optional)
1 tsp turmeric
1 tsp cumin
½ cup currants
3 cups vegetable stock
2 Tbsp chopped fresh parsley
2 Tbsp chopped fresh coriander

½ cup raw pistachio nuts, chopped
Method

Cook the onion and garlic in the oil for 5 minutes. Add the spices and rice, and stir for 1 minute. Add the currants and stock, bring to the boil, then simmer covered for 25-30 minutes, until the rice is cooked, and nearly all the liquid has been absorbed. You will need to stir occasionally. Stir in the chopped parsley and coriander. Serve sprinkled with the pistachio nuts.

Mediterranean Stuffed Capsicums

Serves 4

Ingredients

1 Tbsp olive oil
1 onion, chopped
1 zucchini, diced
1 clove garlic, finely chopped
115g mushrooms, sliced
400g tinned tomatoes, chopped
1 Tbsp tomato paste
1/3 cup pine nuts
2 Tbsp chopped fresh basil
4 large capsicums
1 tsp sweet paprika
Sea salt & black pepper to taste

Method

Preheat the oven to 180 degrees Celsius. Cook the onion, garlic, zucchini and mushrooms in olive oil for 3 minutes. Add the tinned tomatoes and tomato paste. Bring to the boil, then simmer uncovered for 10-15 minutes, until thickened slightly. Remove from the heat, stir in the pine nuts, basil and spices. Cut the capsicums in half lengthways, and remove the seeds. Blanch in boiling water for 3 minutes, then drain well. Place capsicums in a greased oven dish, fill with vegetable mixture and cover with foil. Bake for 20 minutes. Remove the foil and bake a further 5-10 minutes. Serve with brown rice.

Chili Corn Pasta

Serves 4

Ingredients

1 onion, chopped
2 cloves garlic, finely chopped (optional)
1 Tbsp olive oil
1 can tinned tomatoes, chopped
300g tomato paste
½ tsp cayenne powder (optional)
1 tsp cumin
1 tsp turmeric
1 tsp red wine vinegar
1 tin red kidney beans, rinsed & drained
Sea salt & black pepper to taste
1 packet gluten free corn pasta
Fresh basil leaves to garnish

Method

Cook the pasta according to packet directions. Cook the onion and garlic in oil gently for 5 minutes. Add the spices, and then add remaining ingredients except the pasta. Simmer covered for 30 minutes, stirring occasionally. Serve over the pasta; garnish with basil.

Spicy Bean Risotto

Serves 4

Ingredients

1 Tbsp olive oil
1 onion, finely chopped
2 cloves garlic, finely chopped (optional)
5 sun-dried tomatoes (soak in boiling water for ½ hour)
1 cup brown rice
1 Tbsp tomato paste
560mL vegetable stock or water
1 tsp sweet paprika
1 tsp dried coriander powder
1 zucchini, diced
1 bunch English spinach, chopped
1 can navy or lima beans, rinsed & drained

Method

Cook the onion and garlic in oil for 5 minutes. Drain the sun-dried tomatoes and chop. Add the rice to the onion mixture, making sure it is well coated with oil. Add the spices, tomato paste, sun-dried tomatoes and stock. Simmer covered for 15 minutes. Add the zucchini, spinach and beans, and continue cooking for another 20 minutes, or until the rice is cooked. You will need to stir regularly, and add more water if it is required. Serve with a salad.

Chick Pea Curry

Serves 4

Ingredients

1 tin chick peas
1 Tbsp olive oil
1 onion, chopped
2 cloves garlic, finely chopped (optional)
1 Tbsp grated ginger (optional)
2 tsp turmeric
2 tsp cumin
2 tsp sweet paprika
1 tsp curry powder (optional)
1 cup vegetable stock
1 Swede, cubed
2 cups cubed pumpkin
2 button squash, chopped
1 can tinned tomatoes, chopped

Method

Cook the onion, garlic and ginger in oil for 5 minutes. Add the spices and cook a further 2 minutes. Add all the other ingredients except the squash; simmer covered for 20 minutes. Add the squash and simmer a further 10 minutes. Serve with brown rice and garnish with fresh coriander.

Cannellini Bean Patties

Serves 4

Ingredients

2 cups canned cannellini beans
1 carrot, finely diced
¼ onion, finely diced
1 Tbsp chopped parsley
½ cup gluten free rice crumbs, or brown rice flour
2 Tbsp toasted sesame seeds
Lemon juice

Method

Preheat the oven to 180 degrees Celsius. Mash the beans well.
Mix all ingredients together to form patties. If mixture is too dry,
add lemon juice; if it is too moist, add more crumbs or flour.
Brush with olive oil and bake for approximately 30 minutes; until
lightly browned. Serve with a salad.

Tempeh Stir-Fried Rice

You should find tempeh alongside tofu, in the refrigerated section
of supermarkets.

Serves 4

Ingredients

1 Tbsp olive oil
2 cloves garlic, finely chopped (optional)
1 carrot, diced
4 mushrooms, chopped

1 cup cooked green peas
2 cups cooked brown rice
1 packet tempeh
1 Tbsp tamari
1 tsp cumin

Method

Cook the garlic, onion and carrot in oil for 5 minutes. Add
the tempeh and cook a further 3 minutes. Add the remaining
ingredients, mix well and cook for 5 minutes.
Serve with a salad.

Baked Nutty Vegetables

Serves 4

Ingredients

½ onion, finely chopped
2 cloves garlic, chopped (optional)
1 Tbsp olive oil
2 turnips, diced
4 parsnips, diced
3 Tbsp ground almonds or hazelnuts
½ tsp kelp powder (omit if you can't find it)
1 tsp sweet paprika
1 Tbsp tamari
½ cup water

Method

Preheat oven to 180 degrees Celsius. Sauté the onion and garlic
in oil for 2 minutes. Add the turnips and parsnips and cook a
further 5 minutes. Place vegetable mixture in a greased casserole

dish. Combine the remaining ingredients together and pour over vegetables. Bake covered for 30-40 minutes.
Serve with brown rice.

Tofu Stir-Fry

Serves 4

Ingredients

120g tofu, drained & cut into cubes
1 Tbsp olive oil
4 cups chopped broccoli
1 cup snow peas, halved
½ onion, chopped
1 large carrot, thinly sliced
1 red capsicum, sliced
1 Tbsp tamari
1 tsp grated ginger
½ cup water

Method

Heat oil in a wok or large frying pan. Cook tofu, stirring often until it browns lightly. Add ginger and vegetables, stirring constantly. Add water and tamari. Cook until vegetables are tender and water has evaporated.
Serve with brown rice.

Pasta with Pesto Dressing

Serves 4

Ingredients

2 green capsicums, halved & deseeded
¾ cup pepitas (hulled pumpkin seeds)
2 avocados
1 cup fresh coriander, chopped
1/3 cup lime juice
¾ cup water
Sea salt & black pepper to taste
1 packet gluten free pasta

Method

Heat capsicums in the oven, skin side up until the skins are
charred. Once cooled, peel the skin from the capsicums and place
capsicums in a food processor. Toast pepitas in the oven until
they start to pop. Keep an eye on them; make sure they do not
burn. Place pepitas, capsicum, avocados, coriander, lime juice, salt
and pepper and water in the processor. Process until smooth and
creamy.
Cook pasta according to packet directions. Place pasta on serving
plates and toss avocado mixture through it.

Cauliflower Pasta

Serves 4

Ingredients

1 packet gluten free pasta

3 cloves garlic, minced (optional)
½ head of cauliflower, broken up into flowerets and cooked
100g pine nuts
100mL olive oil

Method

Cook the pasta according to packet directions. Cook the garlic and pine nuts in 2 tablespoons of the olive oil for 3 minutes. Add the remaining ingredients, combining well. Serve with a salad.

Mediterranean Pasta with Olives

Serves 4

Ingredients

1 packet gluten free pasta
1 fresh chili, seeded & finely chopped (optional)
150g pitted black olives
1 onion, finely chopped
1 zucchini, chopped
4 small mushrooms, chopped
800g tinned tomatoes, chopped
2 Tbsp olive oil
2 cloves garlic, finely chopped (optional)
Sea salt & black pepper to taste

Method

Cook the pasta according to packet directions. Cook the onion, garlic and chili in the oil until lightly browned. Add the tomatoes, mushrooms, zucchini, olives and seasonings. Simmer covered for approximately 20 minutes. Place pasta on serving plates; top with tomato mixture. Serve with a salad.

Pasta with Herbed Vegetables

Serves 4

Ingredients

1 packet gluten free pasta
1 eggplant, peeled and chopped
1/3 cup olive oil
2 button squash, chopped
1 onion, chopped
1 cup diced pumpkin
2 cloves garlic, minced (optional)
3 very ripe tomatoes, chopped
1 Tbsp fresh basil, chopped
1 tsp dried oregano
Sea salt & black pepper to taste

Method

Cook the pasta according to packet directions. Sauté the onion, garlic and pumpkin in the oil for 5 minutes. Add remaining ingredients, except the pasta, cover and simmer for 25 minutes. Serve the vegetable mixture over warm pasta.

Spicy Vegetables in Coconut Milk

Serves 4

Ingredients

1 onion, chopped
1 fresh chili, seeded & chopped (optional)
2 cloves garlic, minced (optional)
1 Tbsp olive oil
2 Tbsp lime juice

140mL tin coconut milk
1 cup green beans, chopped
1 cup cauliflower, chopped
4 Brussels sprouts, chopped
1 tsp grated ginger

Method

Cook the onion and garlic in a wok or large frying pan, in the olive oil for 5 minutes. Add the chili and lime juice. Add the vegetables and stir fry until just cooked. Add the coconut milk and simmer a further 5 minutes. Serve with brown rice.

Adzuki Beans with Brown Rice

Serves 4

Ingredients

1 ½ cups dried adzuki beans
6 cups water
¼ cup arame seaweed
1 onion, chopped
2 carrots, grated
DRESSING
2 Tbsp flaxseed oil
1 Tbsp grated ginger
1 clove garlic, minced (optional)
1 cup parsley, chopped
2 Tbsp wine vinegar
1 Tbsp tamari
¼ cup lemon juice
Cooked brown rice for serving

Method

Soak the arame in cold water for 15 minutes. Place the adzuki

beans, water and seaweed in a large pot. Bring to the boil, then simmer for 30-35 minutes; until the beans are cooked, yet retain their shape. Chop the seaweed into small pieces. Combine all salad ingredients together, including cooked beans. Combine dressing ingredients and mix well with salad.
Serve with brown rice.

Marinated Tempeh

Serves 2

Ingredients

1 packet tempeh
1 tsp olive oil
1 tsp grated ginger (optional)
1 tsp mustard (optional)
1 Tbsp tamari
2 Tbsp water

Method

Preheat the oven to 180 degrees Celsius. Cut the tempeh into squares or triangles and place into a shallow, greased baking dish. Combine all ingredients except the tempeh, and pour them over the tempeh. Bake covered for 20 minutes, turn over and bake uncovered for another 15 minutes.
Serve with a salad or steamed vegetables.

Herbed Lentils

Serves 4

Ingredients

1 cup canned lentils, drained
¼ cup lemon juice
2 Tbsp olive oil
1 capsicum, diced
4 spring onions, sliced
1 head broccoli, chopped
2 zucchinis, chopped
1 large carrot, sliced
1 tsp dried coriander
Sea salt & black pepper to taste

Method

Steam broccoli, carrot and zucchini until tender. Combine all ingredients together in a large bowl. Can be served on its own or with brown rice.

Bean Spread

Makes 2 cups

Ingredients

2 cups canned Lima or other beans
¼ cup olive oil
3 cloves garlic, crushed (optional)
Juice of 1 lemon
1 tsp sweet paprika
¼ tsp cayenne (optional)

Sea salt & black pepper to taste

Method

Cook the garlic in the oil gently for 3 minutes. Once cooled, place the garlic and beans in a food processor. Process until smooth. With the motor running add the olive oil, lemon juice and seasonings, and process until smooth.
Serve on gluten free toast, rice or corn crackers with a salad.

Quinoa Pilaf

Serves 4

Ingredients

¾ cup quinoa
1 Tbsp olive oil
1 onion, diced
2 cloves garlic, crushed (optional)
2 ½ cups boiling water
1/3 cup currants
¼ cup chopped pecans
1 tsp turmeric
1 tsp cumin
Sea salt & black pepper to taste

Method

Cook the onion and garlic in the oil gently for 3 minutes. Stir in the quinoa and cook a further 3 minutes. Add the boiling water and seasonings. Simmer covered for 20-25 minutes, or until the water has been absorbed. Stir in the currants and pecans, and serve.

Rice with Red Lentils

Serves 3

Ingredients

1 cup red lentils
1 ½ cups water
1 Tbsp olive oil
1 onion, diced
6 cloves garlic, crushed (optional)
1 Tbsp sesame seeds
1 tsp turmeric
1 tsp cumin
¼ tsp cayenne (optional)
Sea salt & black pepper
Cooked brown rice for serving

Method

Soak lentils for 3 hours or longer before cooking. Discard the soaking water, rinse the lentils, and place in a pot with 1 ½ cups fresh water. Add the spices and simmer for approximately 15-20 minutes; until the lentils are soft and pulpy. Add more water if required. Sauté the onion, garlic, sesame seeds, salt and pepper in oil until lightly browned. Stir the onion mixture into the lentils, and serve over brown rice. Serve this with steamed vegetables or a salad.

Adzuki Bean Stew

Serves 4

Ingredients

1 cup adzuki beans
2 cups diced pumpkin
2 cloves garlic, minced (optional)
4 mushrooms, sliced
1 stick celery, sliced
1 piece kombu, washed
1 Tbsp tamari

Method

Soak the beans in water overnight, discard the water and rinse the beans. Put the beans and kombu in a pot and cover with water. Simmer until the beans soften, this takes approximately 20 minutes. Sauté the garlic, pumpkin, mushrooms and celery in oil for 5 minutes. Add the beans, chopped kombu, tamari and ½ cup water to the vegetable mixture. Cook 15 minutes, or until vegetables are cooked and most of the water has evaporated. Serve with a salad.

Baked Borlotti Beans with Rice

Serves 4

Ingredients

1 cup cooked borlotti beans
1 cup cooked brown rice
2 sheets toasted nori, torn into small pieces
½ large sweet potato, diced

1 bunch bok choy, chopped
1 carrot, diced
1 onion, chopped
1 Tbsp olive oil
Sea salt & black pepper
1 block firm tofu
2 Tbsp tahini
Juice of 1 lemon
¼ cup seeded olives
2 Tbsp sesame seeds

Method

Preheat the oven to 180 degrees Celsius. Sauté the onion, salt and pepper in olive oil for 5 minutes. Steam the sweet potato, bok choy and carrot until cooked. Grease a casserole dish and put the cooked rice and beans, and nori pieces on the bottom. Place the cooked onion, sweet potato, bok choy and carrot on top.
Blend the tofu, tahini and lemon juice together in a food processor until smooth. Add more water if required. Put the olives on top of the vegetables, then smooth the tofu paste on top. Sprinkle with sesame seeds.
Bake for 15-20 minutes, until lightly browned.

Black Eyed Beans with Spinach

Serves 2

Ingredients

½ cup black eyed beans
1 clove garlic, crushed (optional)
1 Tbsp olive oil
1 bunch English spinach, chopped
1 red capsicum, chopped finely

1 Tbsp balsamic vinegar
Sea salt & black pepper to taste

Method

Soak the beans in water overnight, discard the water and rinse the beans. Simmer the beans in fresh water until cooked, this will take approximately 30 minutes. Sauté the garlic and capsicum in oil for 5 minutes. Add the cooked beans, spinach, salt and pepper, and cook a further 2 minutes. Serve seasoned with balsamic vinegar.

Spicy Chick Peas

Serves 4

Ingredients

1 onion, diced
2 cloves garlic, crushed (optional)
3 potatoes, diced
½ cup green beans, chopped
½ large eggplant, peeled & chopped
1 tin tomatoes
1 tin chick peas
1 tsp curry powder (optional)
Sea salt & black pepper to taste
150mL vegetable stock, or water

Method

Cook the onion and garlic in oil for 5 minutes. Add the potatoes and seasonings, and cook a further 2 minutes. Add remaining ingredients and simmer covered for approximately 30 minutes. Serve with brown rice.

Chili Beans

Serves 4

Ingredients

1 tin butter or navy beans
1 onion, finely chopped
2 cloves garlic, minced (optional)
1 Tbsp olive oil
1 bunch bok choy, chopped
1 tsp turmeric
½ tsp cayenne powder (optional)
1 tsp sweet paprika
2 tsp tomato paste
1 tin tomatoes, chopped
1 cup vegetable stock
1 tsp arrowroot flour

Method

Cook the onion and garlic in oil for 5 minutes. Add all other ingredients except arrowroot. Simmer for 15 minutes. Mix the arrowroot with a little cold water to form a paste. Stir well into the chili mixture, and continue cooking a few minutes until it thickens to the desired level.
Serve with brown rice and a salad.

Detox Shepherd's Pie

Serves 4

Ingredients

1 cup brown lentils
1 tsp sweet paprika
½ tsp cayenne (optional)
1 Tbsp olive oil
2 cloves garlic, crushed (optional)
1 onion, chopped
1 cup mushrooms, sliced
1 large zucchini, chopped
1 red capsicum, chopped
1 head broccoli, chopped
1 Tbsp tamari
¾ cup vegetable stock
4 Tbsp tomato paste
2 ½ cups mashed potato

Method

Soak the lentils overnight, drain and rinse them. Preheat the oven
to 200 degrees Celsius.
Cook the lentils in a pot of fresh water for approximately 15
minutes, or until they soften. Drain the lentils and set aside.
Sauté the onion, garlic and mushrooms in oil for 5 minutes. Add
the remaining vegetables and sauté for 5 more minutes.
Add the remaining ingredients, except the mashed potato. Simmer
for 8-10 minutes, until thickened. Place the mixture into a
casserole dish and top with mashed potato. Cook in the oven for
15 minutes, or until browned.
Serve with salad.

Tomato Pasta Casserole

Serves 6

Ingredients

800g tinned tomatoes
1 cup tomato paste
1 onion, chopped
2 cloves garlic, crushed (optional)
1 Tbsp olive oil
1 bunch baby bok choy, chopped
1 cup chopped, pitted black olives
800g tinned kidney beans
1 tsp dried oregano
1 tsp sweet paprika
Sea salt & black pepper to taste
2 Tbsp chopped fresh basil
1 packet gluten free pasta, cooked

Method

Preheat the oven to 180 degrees Celsius.
Cook the garlic and onion in the oil for 5 minutes. Add all
remaining ingredients except the pasta. Simmer for 20 minutes.
Mix bean mixture with the pasta and place in a casserole dish.
Bake for 20 minutes at 180 degrees Celsius.

Salad Dressing Recipes

You may use the dressings provided in the salad recipes which start on page 157, make up your own, or use the ones below. It is fine to use no dressing at all.

Italian Dressing

Ingredients

1 cup cold pressed olive oil
1 clove garlic, minced (optional)
½ cup lemon juice
½ tsp dried oregano

Place all ingredients into a sealed jar and shake well. Store in the refrigerator.

Vinegar Dressing

Ingredients

½ cup balsamic or red wine vinegar
½ cup cold pressed olive oil
2 tsp tamari

Place all ingredients into a sealed jar and shake well. Store in the refrigerator.

Hummus Dressing

Ingredients

Juice of 2 lemons
3 Tbsp hummus

1 clove garlic, minced (optional)
1 Tbsp cold pressed olive oil

Place all ingredients into a sealed jar; stir with a fork and then shake well. Store in the refrigerator.

Zesty Dressing

Ingredients

¼ cup lime juice
1 tsp grated lime zest
1 tsp grated fresh ginger
½ cup cold pressed walnut oil (or olive oil)

Place all ingredients into a sealed jar and shake well. Store in the refrigerator.

Salad Recipes

Quinoa Tabouli

You should find quinoa in the health isle of a good supermarket, or in a health food store. Rice can be used in its place.

Serves 3

Ingredients

1 cup quinoa
2 cups water
Sea salt & black pepper to taste
½ cup frozen peas
1 tomato, diced
1 stalk celery, finely chopped
10 olives, sliced
Large handful parsley, finely chopped
Large handful chives, finely chopped
Juice of ½ lemon

Method

Simmer the quinoa in the water, salt and pepper approximately 20 minutes, or until cooked and all water has evaporated. Blanch the peas for one minute. Mix all ingredients together in a large bowl. Serve.

Rena's Red Kohl rabi Salad

Serves 3

Ingredients

2 medium kohlrabi, peeled and grated
1 cup grated raw beetroot
1 red capsicum, sliced thinly
¼ cup chopped fresh coriander
1 tsp grated ginger
Flaxseed oil and lemon juice for dressing

Method

Combine vegetables together in a bowl. Combine ginger, oil and lemon juice together and pour over salad.

Cucumber Salad

Serves 2

Ingredients

1 Lebanese cucumber, sliced
1/2 red onion, sliced
2 Tbsp chopped fresh basil
2 radishes, sliced
1 carrot, coarsely grated
Flaxseed oil & red wine vinegar as dressing

Method

Mix salad ingredients together in a bowl and pour dressing on top.

Garden Salad with Avocado Dressing

Serves 3

Ingredients

1 cucumber, sliced
1 tomato, diced
2 button mushrooms, sliced
1 carrot, finely sliced
Radicchio lettuce, shredded
DRESSING
1 avocado
Juice of ½ lemon
½ cup water
1 tsp chopped fresh dill
Sea salt & black pepper to taste

Method

Combine the salad ingredients together and arrange on plates.
Blend the dressing ingredients together until smooth. Pour
dressing over salad.

Chick Pea and Broccoli Salad

Serves 4

Ingredients

1 can chick peas, drained
2 cups lightly cooked broccoli
½ red onion, sliced
½ cup snow peas, halved
1 carrot, sliced thinly

Sea salt & black pepper to taste
DRESSING
2 Tbsp flaxseed oil
3 Tbsp tahini
1 clove garlic, minced (optional)
1 ½ Tbsp lemon juice
2 Tbsp tamari
3 Tbsp water
Method

Blend dressing ingredients together until smooth. Combine salad ingredients together with dressing and serve.

Carrot Salad

Makes 4 cups

Ingredients

3 cups grated carrot
4 radishes, thinly sliced
1 stalk celery, thinly sliced
½ cup currants
¼ cup lemon juice
2 Tbsp olive oil
Sea salt & black pepper to taste

Method

Combine ingredients together and serve.

Nutty Chick Pea Salad

Serves 4

Ingredients

2 cups cooked chick peas
¼ cup freshly roasted pecans
4 spring onions, thinly sliced
1 cup grated daikon (white) radish (use carrot if unavailable)
1 cup grated beetroot
¼ cup coriander, finely chopped
2 Tbsp olive oil
¼ cup lemon juice
1 Tbsp tamari

Method

Combine ingredients together and serve.

Avocado Salad

Serves 4

Ingredients

1 avocado, sliced
4 radishes, sliced
4 spring onions, sliced
8 cherry tomatoes, sliced
2 Tbsp chopped fresh parsley
10 raw cashew nuts
1 clove garlic, crushed (optional)
Flaxseed oil & lemon juice as dressing
Method
Combine salad ingredients together. Dress with oil, lemon juice
and crushed garlic.

Winter Vegetable Salad

Serves 4

Ingredients

½ bunch chicory, torn into pieces
1 cup coriander, finely chopped
1 cooked parsnip, chopped
2 cooked carrots, diced
1 cooked turnip, diced
½ cup toasted walnuts
DRESSING
2 Tbsp walnut oil (use flaxseed if unavailable)
1 clove garlic, crushed (optional)
½ cup apple cider vinegar
¼ tsp stevia powder, or 1 drop liquid stevia

Method

Arrange salad ingredients on serving plates. Combine dressing ingredients together in a screw-top jar and shake. Pour dressing over salad.

Avocado and Sunflower Salad

Serves 2

Ingredients

1 avocado, sliced
1 tomato, chopped
1 Tbsp finely chopped basil
1 Tbsp apple cider vinegar
Radicchio lettuce, torn
2 Tbsp freshly toasted sunflower seeds

Method

Arrange lettuce leaves on a serving plate. Arrange remaining ingredients on top of lettuce, and lastly sprinkle with sunflower seeds.

Rice and Sesame Salad

Serves 4

Ingredients

2 cups cooked brown rice
½ cup snow peas, halved
1 red capsicum, diced
2 Tbsp chopped walnuts
DRESSING
1 Tbsp Balsamic vinegar
1 clove garlic, crushed (optional)
1 Tbsp toasted sesame seeds
1 Tbsp tamari

Method

Mix salad ingredients together. Combine dressing ingredients and mix well with salad.

Mixed Bean Salad

Serves 4

Ingredients
1 tin three or four bean mix
2 sticks celery, finely chopped
1 green capsicum, finely diced
4 radishes, sliced
2 Tbsp chopped parsley
4 spring onions, finely chopped
Olive oil & lemon juice as dressing

Method

Combine all ingredients and mix well. Serve with brown rice or gluten free pasta.

Bean and Pasta Salad

Serves 4

Ingredients

1 cup tinned kidney beans, rinsed & drained
1 cup cooked gluten free pasta
3 green spring onions, finely chopped
1 punnet cherry tomatoes, halved
1 Tbsp finely chopped parsley
DRESSING
1 Tbsp olive oil
1 Tbsp Balsamic vinegar
1 clove garlic, crushed (optional)
1 tsp mustard

Method

Mix the salad ingredients together in a bowl. Combine the dressing ingredients together in a screw-top jar and shake well. Pour dressing over the salad and serve.

Scary Superbugs are on the rise

Many dangerous and potentially lethal bacteria are now resistant to antibiotics and this huge problem is set to increase. This is for several reasons –

- Antibiotics have been overused in medicine and in food production
- People are very mobile and this spreads antibiotic resistant bacteria rapidly from one side of the world to the other

Bacteria that are resistant to antibiotics carry genes that neutralise the effects of antibiotics, so that these genes make the bacteria indestructible – this is scary stuff!

Bacteria can share and transfer these genes amongst each other and this spreads the antibiotic-resistant genes rapidly across different species of bacteria. In 1991 there were 15 known genes with antibiotic resistance and now there are more than 89.

The consequences of these new resistant genes are –
The re-emergence of tuberculosis
Lethal hospital acquired golden staph infections
Resistant cholera, gonorrhoea, meningitis, pneumonia, gangrene and other severe infections
Longer recovery times for patients with infections

In Britain golden staph caused more than 7600 infections in 2003 and more than 5000 people in Britain died from hospital acquired staph infections.

"Golden staph" stands for the bacteria called staphylococcus aureus and it is commonly resistant to most antibiotics, especially penicillin, which makes it very dangerous, especially in hospitals. Golden staph is commonly found on the skin and in the nasal cavities and is easily spread between people.

Drug companies have realised that antibiotics have a limited future because of increasing bacterial resistance against them, and these drug companies have decided to put far less funding into the development of new antibiotics.

Thus it is vitally important that we turn back to using the natural antibiotics found in nature, as bacteria cannot easily develop resistance against them. Furthermore they are safe and tend to strengthen the immune system and can be used on a long term basis.

Techniques you can use to reduce your exposure to dangerous bacteria are –

Keep your immune system strong by following a healthy diet

Use tea tree oil soap, shampoo and creams on your skin if you or family members have skin infections. Those with infections in the nose and sinuses can use tea tree oil steam inhalations –

Place 2 drops of tea tree oil in a bowl of hot water, place a towel over the head and inhale for 15 minutes. Tea tree oil is a very effective powerful long term anti-septic and can reduce the spread of golden staph.

Take regular supplements of vitamin C and selenium to keep your bacteria-fighting white cells healthy

Use foods with antibiotic properties in your diet – these include garlic, red onions, horseradish, all types of radishes, citrus fruits, capsicums, ginger root, turmeric, chilli, curry and other hot spices. Avoid the overuse or unnecessary use of antibiotic drugs in yourself and your family – remember that antibiotics do nothing to help the common cold or influenza. Use probiotics such as plain acidophilus yogurt, which maintains a healthy population of bacteria in the intestines.

Olive leaf extract has proven antibiotic properties against viruses, bacteria and parasites and is thus helpful to fight a wide range of micro-organisms; olive leaf extract is available in a potent capsule form containing 35mg of standardised oleuropein in each capsule

Use a powerful detox-formula to –

     Keep the bacterial population in your gut healthy

     Keep your liver healthy

     Keep your lymphatic system strong

     Fight infection generally

The best herbs for this purpose are Barberry, Wormwood and Thyme; these are found in the correct dosage in certain formulas such as "Digestive 1-2-3 DETOX-SLIM"

The 1-2-3 principle is explained by the actions of the 3 herbs –
Barberry works on the liver and bowel
Wormwood works on the bowel
Thyme works on the lymphatic system
It is important to use products which contain the correct dosages of these herbs otherwise you will find that symptoms recur within several weeks of stopping the herbs. For more information on detoxifying foods, herbs and supplements phone the Sandra Cabot Health Advisory Service on 02 4655 8855.

Avoid the overuse of sugar in the diet, as it feeds the growth of bacteria and fungi, especially in overweight persons and diabetics. Use stevia or xylitol instead of sugar.

References

Ref. 1 The Australian, 24th March 2004.

Ref. 2 Bioceuticals seminar manual: New Developments in Functional Toxicology and Gastrointestinal Rehabilitation, 2002

Ref. 3 Nature, Air Fresheners Cause a Stink, 10 May, 2004

Ref. 4 & 5 Dept of Water Resources, Victoria. Strategy to Upgrade Drinking Water in Victoria, 1985

Ref. 6 www.mydr.com.au

Ref. 7 www.miessence.com.au

Ref. 8 Arylamine exposures and bladder cancer risk. Yu MC, Skipper PL, Tannenbaum SR, Chan KK, Ross RK. Mutat Res. 2002 Sep 30;506-507:21-8

Ref. 9 Environmental Working Group

Ref. 10 www.fedupwithfoodadditives.org

Ref. 11 Dunne C, O'Mahony L, Murphy L, Thornton G, Morrissey D, O'Halloran S, Feeney M, Flynn S, Fitzgerald G, Daly C, Kiely B, O'Sullivan GC, Shanahan F, Collins JK. In vitro selection criteria for probiotic bacteria of human origin: correlation with in vivo findings. Am J Clin Nutr 2001 Feb;73(2 Suppl):386S-392S.

Ref. 12 Mai V, Morris JG Jr. Colonic bacterial flora: changing understandings in the molecular age. J Nutr 2004 Feb;134(2):459-64

Ref. 13. Carli P et al. Presse Med 1995;24:606-610.

Ref. 14 Altern Med Rev 2000 Apr;5(2):175-7

Ref. 15 Berberine inhibits intestinal secretory response of Vibrio cholerae and Escherichia coli enterotoxins. Sack RB, Froehlich JL. Infect Immun. 1982 Feb; 35(2): 471-475

Ref. 16 Pharmacol Ther 2001 May-Jun; 90(2-3):261-5

Ref. 17 Antimicrobial activity of the essential oils of Thymus vulgaris L. measured using a bioimpedometric method. Marino M, Bersani C, Comi G. J Food Prot. 1999 Sep; 62(9):1017-23.

Ref. 18 Tabak M, Armon R, Potasman I, Neeman I. "In Vitro Inhibition of Helicobacter pylori by Extracts of Thyme". Journal of Applied Bacteriology 1996;80(6):667-72.

Ref. 19 Muto S, et. al. Inhibition by green tea catechins of metabolic activation of procarcinogens by human cytochrome P450. Mutat Res 2001;479(1-2):197-206.

Ref. 20 Akimoto K, et. al. Protective effects of sesamin against liver damage caused by alcohol or carbon tetrachloride in rodents. Ann Nutr Metab 1993;37(4):218-24

Ref. 21 Kassie F. Effects of garden and water cress juices and their constituents, benzyl and phenethyl isothiocyanates, towards benzo(a)pyrene-induced DNA damage: a model study with the single cell gel electrophoresis/Hep G2 assay. Chemico-Biological Interactions 2003;142:285-296.

Ref. 22 Dinkova-Kostova AT. Relation of structure of curcumin analogues to their potencies as inducers of phase 2 detoxification enzymes. Carcinogenesis. 1999;20(5):911-914.

Ref. 23 Wheeler MD, et. al. Glycine: a new anti inflammatory immunonutrient. Cell Mol Life Sci. 1999 Nov 30;56(9-10):843-56.

Ref. 24 Obinata K, Maruyama T, Hayashi M, Watanabe T, Nittono H. Effect of taurine on the fatty liver of children with simple obesity. Adv Exp Med Biol. 1996;403:607-13

Ref. 25 The Journal of Urology December 2001;166:2034-2038.

Ref. 26 Atherosclerosis, Thrombosis, and Vascular Biology, December 2000; 20: 2677-2681

Ref. 27 Antimicrobial properties of allicin from garlic. Ankri S, Mirelman D. Microbes Infect. 1999 Feb;1(2):125-9.

Ref. 28 Ritchason, J., Olive Leaf Extract – Potent Antibacterial, Antiviral and Antifungal Agent, Woodland Publishing Inc., PO Box 160, Pleasant Grove, Utah 84062, 1999

Ref. 29 Gard, Zane R. "Literature Review and Comparison Studies of Sauna/Hyperthermia in Detoxification"

Ref. 30 Zhonghua Yi Xue Za Zhi. 2003 Oct 25;83(20):1764-8 [Analysis of anti-proliferation of curcumin on human breast cancer cells and its mechanism] Breast Surgery Department of Cancer Hospital, Fudan University, Shanghai 200032, China.

Ref. 31 The Curry Spice Curcumin Reduces Oxidative Damage and Amyloid Pathology in an Alzheimer Transgenic Mouse. Lim GP, Chu T, Yang F, Beech W, Frautschy SA, Cole GM.

Departments of Medicine and Neurology, University of California, Los Angeles, Los Angeles, California 90095, and Greater Los Angeles Veterans Affairs Healthcare System, Geriatric Research, Education and Clinical Center, Sepulveda, California 91343.
Ref.32 Paul Pitchford, Healing With Whole Foods: Asian Traditions and Modern Nutrition, North Atlantic Books, 2002.

Immune System References

Dietary Selenium: Time to act, The British Medical Journal, Vol. 314, February 1997
Effects of selenium supplementation for cancer prevention in patients with carcinoma of the skin, Journal American Medical Association, Dec 1996, Vol. 276, no 24
Meydani SN. et al, Vitamin E supplementation and in vivo immune response in healthy elderly subjects. JAMA. 1997; 277:1380-6
Russo MW. et al, Plasma selenium levels and the risk of colorectal adenomas. Nutr Cancer 1997; 28:125-9
Knekt P. et al, Serum selenium, serum vitamin E, and the risk of rheumatoid arthritis. Epidemiology 2000; 11:402-5
Flat A. et al, Reduced selenium in asthmatic subjects in New Zealand. Thorax. 1990; 45:95-9
Clark LC. et al, Effects of selenium supplementation for cancer prevention in patients with carcinoma of the skin. A randomized controlled trial. JAMA. 1996;276:1957-63
Markin D. et al, In vitro antimicrobial activity of olive leaves. Mycoses 2003 April; 46(3-4): 132 -6 (ISSN: 0933-7407)
Lee-Huang S. et al, Anti-HIV activity of olive leaf extract (OLE) and modulation of host cell gene expression by HIV-1 infection and OLE treatment. Biochem Biophys Res Commun 2003 August 8; 307(4):1029-37 (ISSN: 0006-291X)
Bisignano G et al, On the in-vitro antimicrobial activity of oleuropein and hydroxytyrosol. J Pharm Pharmacol 1999 Aug; 51(8):971-4 (ISSN: 0022-3573)
Wang W. et al, Protein extraction for two dimensional electrophoresis of olive leaf, a plant tissue containing high levels of interfering compounds. Electrophoresis (Germany), Jul 2003,

24(14) p2369-75

Briante R. et al, Olea europaea leaf extract and derivatives: antioxidant properties. J Agric Food Chem (USA), Aug 14 2002, 50(17) p4934-40

Renis H E. In vitro antiviral activity of calcium olenolate. Antimicrobial Agents & Chemotherapy, 1970, pp. 167-171

Kaij-a-Kamb, M. et al, Search for new anti-viral agents of plant origin. Pharma-Acta-Helv, 67(5-6): 130-147, 1992

De Whalley, C V. et al, Olive Leaf extract, Biochem Pharmacology 39: 1743-1750, 1990

Elliot G A. et al, Preliminary safety studies with calcium elenolate, an anti-viral agent. Antimicrobial agents and Chemotherapy, 173-176, 1969

Parker, M S. et al, Canadian Journal of Microbiology 141:745-746, 1968

Tranter et al. The effect of the olive phenolic compound, oleuropein, on growth and enterotoxin B production by staph aureus. Journal of Applied Bacteriology 74:253-259, 1993

Walker M. Antimicrobial attributes of olive leaf extract, Townsend Letter for doctors and patients, #156, July 1996, pp.80-85

Rodriguez M. et al, Olive leaf, Journal of Applied Bacteriology 64; 219-225, 1988

The Detox Box – nature's most powerful force for clearing toxic overload

Detoxification is essential in our modern age of technological sophistication and complex pollutants. We simply can't avoid the vast array of chemical and electrical pollutants so we need to maintain our toxicity below the point at which disease symptoms appear. An accumulation of toxins can be disastrous to our health and may result in a variety of disease labels such as arthritis, heart disease, cancer, Parkinson's Disease and Chronic Fatigue Syndrome to name a few. The answer to reducing our toxic load is in developing an effective detoxification program. When detoxifying, we must not overlook the detoxification pathways of our largest organ, the skin. Toxins can be expelled through the skin in sweat. This effective method works in synergy with what may be an already over worked liver and allows our body to expel a greater amount of toxins.

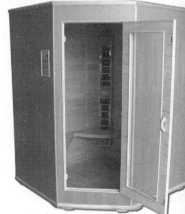

A new form of sweating therapy has been introduced to Australia after success in Europe, Japan and the USA. Far infrared rays have been applied to a cabin, warming the user with only gentle heating of the air. The air is warm and dry, compared to the super-heated air of the traditional saunas. This new 'smart' far infrared sauna is comfortable and particularly well tolerated by sufferers of illness including end-stage heart disease.

History

Sweating therapy has long been recognised as an effective way to reduce the severity of illness and maintain good health.

The Ultimate Detox

Applications have evolved in many cultures however the health benefits still continue to impress, surviving hundreds of years of advancement in medicine. The Native American Indians introduced sweat lodges and Traditional Chinese Medicine encourages the taking of herbal preparations and hot baths. In Sweden and Turkey, heat and steam based saunas have long been enjoyed for their health giving properties. Often it is people who suffer from illness and heart conditions that react most adversely to extreme heat, so the idea of gaining any of the benefits of sweating therapy is completely out of the question for these people. Regrettably, these people stand to gain the most. So low temperature far infrared sauna is a welcome solution in the treatment of such conditions.

How it works

Far infrared rays are safe and naturally occur as part of the sun's light spectrum. Very different from harmful ultraviolet rays that burn the skin, far infrared rays have been used in the NASA space program to assist astronauts to maintain cardiovascular fitness and even in humidicribs to warm premature babies. We feel the effects of infrared as the deep warmth that we get from the sun on an early winter's morning.

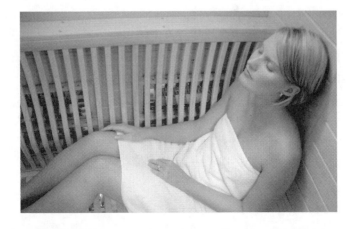

This smart technology uses far infrared rays to heat the body deeply (up to 6cms below the skin) to induce a high volume of sweat (2-3 times as much as a traditional sauna and with a higher proportion of toxins). The temperature is a very comfortable 40-50°C.

Benefits

We expect a range of benefits from using this far infrared technology on a regular basis.

- Detoxify safely and effectively

Many of today's toxins and heavy metals have been difficult to remove from the body. They are bound in the fat layer below the skin. This technology enables us to sweat the toxins from the body, even heavy metals such as mercury and lead.

- Energise the body and relax the mind

We notice a great sense of relaxation and revitalisation as our body releases endorphins, the happy drug. Researchers have linked it to enhancing the immune system, relieving pain, reducing stress and delaying the aging process.

- Clear cellulite

Research shows that cellulite becomes water soluble at 43°C. This gel-like substance comprises fat, water and waste products and can be sweated away. When combined with massage and diet, the results are even greater.

- Improve skin tone

Studies have shown that the gentle far infrared rays support cell energy. This in turn improves the look and function of our skin. Lesley Kenton says, in her best-selling book Skin Revolution, "Nature's most powerful force for clearing toxic overload, it is also an effective and delightful method for healing, regenerating and rejuvenating the skin."

- Assist in weight management

Far infrared waves can help to trigger fat burning, clearing out of lipophilic toxins stored in the body's fat cells. Once the store of these pollutants has been diminished, weight loss becomes an easier process. Using this far infrared technology, it is possible to burn up to 600 calories in just one 30-minute session.

What to look for

In Australia, far infrared saunas are starting to appear in medical clinics and health centres, however the most economical way to use this therapy is probably to buy one for your own home. Dr Rogers writes in Detoxify or Die, "I used to hesitate to recommend something as expensive as a home sauna. I was looking for treatments that were natural but inexpensive and definitely not high tech! But when you realize the lifelong incapacity and expense of diseases such as chronic pain syndromes, heart disease, chemical sensitivity, chronic fatigue, fibromyalgia, migraines, Alzheimer's, cancer or any others caused by chemical toxicity, a sauna is cheap. Let's face it: high-tech pollution requires high-tech solutions." When using the far infrared sauna for health reasons it is essential to check that the timber used is hypoallergenic such as spruce or poplar.

The Detox Box, a well-names far infrared technology designed by Australian company High Tech Health, is the far infrared sauna of choice by many high profile health practitioners. It is constructed from Russian spruce timber, with the use of non-toxic glues. Several high quality ceramic bar heaters are placed strategically within the unit to produce optimal far infrared rays. Five standard models range in size from the one-person cabinet to the four-person cabin. The Detox Box includes conveniences such as CD Player, air ioniser and both internal and external controls.

Far infrared therapy is safe, comfortable, convenient, affordable and effective. We need to incorporate it into our daily lives to counter the long-term toxic effects of the modern environment from which none of us can escape. With proven results in removing heavy metals and toxins, improving skin tone, controlling weight conditions and simply maintaining good health, this relatively new technology is an essential health tool for achieving and maintaining good health. If you are serious about gaining optimum health, then make sure to include regular far infrared sauna sessions in your program.

Contact

High Tech Health
Ph: 1800 505 108
www.hightechhealth.com.au
info@hightechhealth.com.au

Detox your body and save your health

The Art and Science of Iridology

By Clinical Nutritionist Sheree Ward
Phone: 02 4655 8855

The eyes are not just the window to the soul but provide a window to help the practitioner of iridology to discover underlying imbalances in the body.

Iridology (also known as iris diagnosis) is a safe non-invasive and useful health assessment tool which can be dated back to the time of Hippocrates. Today, it is widely used by trained iridologists to help pinpoint the cause of health problems and imbalances in the body.

Iridology can be helpful in determining the causes of symptoms and conditions such as –
- Emotional and mental imbalances
- Inflammation
- Congestion in the lymphatic system
- Liver dysfunction
- Kidney dysfunction
- Digestive and bowel problems

It can also check the body's constitution such as hidden strengths and weaknesses that are genetically determined.

Body toxicity can be assessed by the changes in the pattern of the iris. These can be found in the colours, marks and signs in the iris, which mirror specific parts of the body's organs and systems.

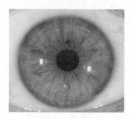 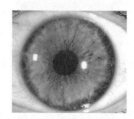 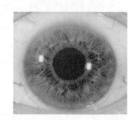

This complementary assessment tool assists the iridologist in determining the cause of current ill health, guiding you to managing future optimum health.

Is Detoxification What You Need?

Detox and restore your immune system

Do you suffer with -:

- ☐ **A weak immune system**
- ☐ **Frequent infections**
- ☐ **Headaches**
- ☐ **Bowel problems**
- ☐ **Bad breath**
- ☐ **Skin problems**
- ☐ **Weight excess**

IF YOU TICKED ANY OF THE ABOVE, YOU NEED IRIS ASSESSMENT AND DR CABOT'S NEW TWO WEEK CLEANSING DIET NOW!

To book your iris analysis and iris photo,
Call our iridologists at our Camden Clinic (02) 4655 4666
We use the latest state of the art computerized iris camera.

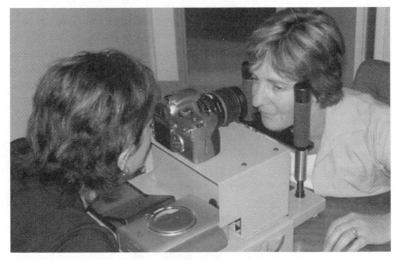

Dr Sandra Cabot's Natural Hormone and Weight Loss Clinics
www.whas.com.au – for free on line
Dr Cabot Health Newsletters

The Most Advanced Wellness Filter Ever Produced

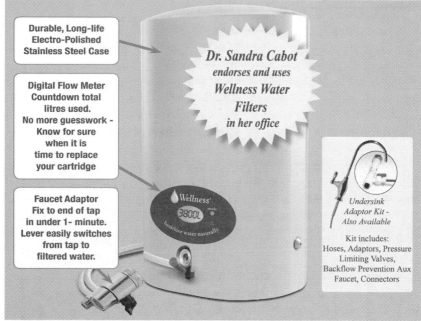

Durable, Long-life Electro-Polished Stainless Steel Case

Digital Flow Meter Countdown total litres used. No more guesswork - Know for sure when it is time to replace your cartridge

Faucet Adaptor Fix to end of tap in under 1- minute. Lever easily switches from tap to filtered water.

Dr. Sandra Cabot endorses and uses Wellness Water Filters in her office

Undersink Adaptor Kit - Also Available

Kit includes:
Hoses, Adaptors, Pressure Limiting Valves, Backflow Prevention Aux Faucet, Connectors

---

Naturally, when drinking water we want to be certain in the knowledge that common contaminants such as dirt, rust and sediment have been removed. Wellness is designed with this thought in mind.

However, removing gross contaminants is only the first step towards a healthy water. After all, who wants to drink chlorine, chemicals and other nasties that have been routinely linked to increased risks of disease?

Our goal is always to bring you more than just good water, we want to give you outstanding water.

Water that tastes great and feels as if it has just come from the freshest, most pure and healthiest mountain spring on earth.

Wellness brings water back to life. How?

Enhancing Water

Starting with a base of healthy water we now 'enhance' your water. In this patented process rare volcanic minerals, synergistically combined over multiple layers, do more than just improve taste.

These layers work just like a natural mountain spring to make the healthiest water available today. The Wellness Filter;

- *Retains beneficial minerals*
- *Elutes micro traces magnesium*
- *Stabilises and balances pH*
- *Improves water solubility*
- *Imparts healthy far-infrared energy*

This scientifically proven process not only improves the taste and texture of water it also affects important energetic changes and makes Wellness the most sought after and endorsed water in the world.

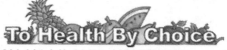

To Health By Choice

Freecall: Aust - 1800 021 069 N.Z. - 0800 726 766 www.tohealth.com.au

---

The Ultimate Detox

Cholesterol: The Real Truth
Discover the real cause of
heart disease

A ground breaking NEW BOOK by Dr Sandra Cabot and naturopath Margaret Jasinska.
To be released mid 2005

Learn about:

■ The dangers of cholesterol lowering drugs

■ The scam of pushing cholesterol drugs - it's a profit driven industry, not health care in YOUR best interests

■ Lowering cholesterol could ruin your sex life

■ Lowering cholesterol could ruin your memory

■ Lowering cholesterol could make you miserable and depressed

■ Should cholesterol be as low as possible? - scare tactics exposed

■ Natural treatments to lower cholesterol - safe and as effective as drugs

■ Foods to lower cholesterol

■ The real cause of heart disease – inflammation is at the root of heart disease

■ The hidden risk factors for heart disease exposed – learn which tests you MUST have

■ Juice recipes & Soup recipe to lower cholesterol

The Ultimate Detox